TABLE OF CONTENTS

The

Sacred Language

Of The

Human Body

By Mona Delfino

Dedicated to the Memory

of Dr. John Jay Harper

and to the Healing of Humanity

~ Acknowledgements ~

I would like to dedicate this book to everyone who ever touched my life, came across my path, and smiled at me in a public place without knowing who I was. I dedicate it to Spirit, the source of this book, and to everyone it reaches. You, the reader, are precious to me. If it weren't for you, the world would be a little less curious, a little less caring, and a little less wise. Therefore, you are the star of the show.

My gratitude goes out to all of those who have supported me in writing my first book. I am grateful to my 5,000 friends on Facebook and Twitter, who have read my posts daily and are still my friends!

My mentor who is gone from this world, Karen Land, deserves to be acknowledged for all of the 12 years I spent learning from this wise Cherokee healer.

To my kids, Leah, Rachel, and Joshua, who have always been my best friends.

To my sisters, Donna, Lucy, and Cindy, who knew I was a weird little kid and loved me anyway.

To all my loved ones who have crossed over into the other worlds. I love you and know you are here and there.

To my dog Kita, who saved my life on December 15, 2010, and to my deaf cat, Maya, who makes up for her deafness by making me listen to her twice as much.

I want to thank Dr. Bernie Siegel, one of my dearest heroes throughout my life, who spoke similar words of wisdom in the '80's when he was working so hard as a medical doctor, doing his best to tell the truth of life everywhere he went to all the people he touched. He still does. He touched my heart.

To Dr. Norm Shealy, another fabulous man who, as a neurosurgeon, understood that we all need each other to heal. How blessed we are to have these incredible heroes in our world!

My editors, Sue Kay and Barbara Stott, thank you for asking me to take out all the little dots that became habit forming during the course of writing this book, and of course, for all your support!

I want to acknowledge my dear friend and client, Leslie Ruchala, a beautiful lady who taught me how to write a book. Being from Jersey, thank goodness she holds absolutely nothin' back.

Doug Cristafir is one of the most talented Graphic Artists known to man, woman, and every alien in the Universe! I have him to thank for the amazing book cover, my business cards, and my website. (Did I mention putting together this book as well?)

Last but not least, I dedicate this book to Pele, the Goddess of Hawaii. She taught me how to listen to the wind, watch, learn, and live the magic of Aloha. She had her own courage to request a part in the book in 2009 because she loves people and wanted them to understand that love is what grows our world. Her fire purifies the heart of man, as she is truly a Goddess.

Thank you, everybody. Now, let's get this party started!

~ About the Author ~

I am Mona Delfino, a Shaman by birth and overall a very happy healer. As a medical intuitive, energy runner, and healer for the last 30 years, I feel that putting this book out today is crucial with the amount of people I see shifting into who they truly are. In some ways, we might say this is a book of "Life 101" for people who are beginning to see themselves and every person around them going through immense change. In this book I will share with you a few experiences of when I was a kid so you can see that, from the beginning, these teachings are from absolute truth from my heart to yours.

All of the thousands of healings I have contributed to have made such differences in these people that I feel *now* is the time to share this knowledge of how energy healing works. As far as I can see, this is what the future of health care is truly about, and it may provide answers to many questions arising around this dynamic topic. My feeling is strong about helping people discover their soul's true nature.

I am skilled and certified in sound therapy; however, I feel the intent of the human voice is the best sound therapist. I have studied and had many opportunities to learn Indigenous ways, Native American and Hawaiian as well, along with several types of medicinal techniques.

My love for the Indigenous began when I went on a trip to Pago Pago, American Samoa, in 1974. I was 16 years old when I sang and traveled with a musical group from Oceanside, California. We did a lot of performing; however, the day we were asked to perform in our Sister City, Pago Pago, I felt like my world was complete!

There were about 20 of us kids, and the second day we were invited to something very special. We were told that we would be going to see the home of an elderly lady and her granddaughter; both had passed away many years prior. Little did I know when we arrived by bus to this house overlooking a very steep cliff, that this would be the adventure that started me on my way into healing and passion for the Indigenous for the rest of my life.

When we arrived and were still on the bus, we were told the story of the turtle and the shark. I remember being mesmerized by the beautiful tropical area on this gorgeous terrain as our tour guide spoke gently of the granddaughter's and the elderly lady's eventual demise. She said that the two of them had told each other that if one were to die, the other would soon follow. The little girl wanted to be a turtle, and the grandmother told her she would be the shark. It was a type of contract that they set up. One day it happened. The little girl was playing on the nearby cliff when she slipped and fell into the ocean about 200 feet down. The grandmother saw her fall and jumped soon afterwards to her death as well.

The tour guide explained the importance of respect. She told us that anyone who yelled loudly or became disruptive would stop the magic of what was to come. I was intrigued! She also told us that if we pointed our fingers or used a camera, we would be sadly disappointed. So off we went onto the land to the area of where the cliff met its end and where the ocean waves crashing on the rocks below had me hooked.

—
8

The guide began to sing in Samoan a beautiful song, "Malieh Telifah," and was throwing rose petals into the water far below to lure the shark and the turtle to come see us. At this point my eyes must have been as big as saucers. Then it happened. The turtle showed up first in the waves as we gazed below. Within five minutes, the shark appeared with the fin showing, then making a little jump as it circled the turtle. It was breathtaking. I was in shock as I watched the most amazing thing I had ever witnessed. My heart felt as though it stopped beating.

Then one of the kids in our singing group pointed her finger and said, "There they are!" The turtle and the shark both went under the water and never came back up that we could see. The tour guide was absolutely correct. I was so amazed I didn't even have the urge to throw the girl who pointed over the cliff! From that day on, my life was changed. I would memorize that song and keep the memory always in my heart. That was a myth or legend that was told in Samoa, and here we were so fortunate to see it as reality.

That same trip I developed a fever and almost died with a 106 degree temperature. Needless to say, our one week of singing became the trip of a lifetime for me, and I would never be the same. My life began taking shape from there.

As I was finishing high school, I was also blessed to have been well received in another singing group called The Young Americans, which I was a part of for two years. When I turned 18, I received my first calling from Spirit. It was a feeling so undeniably strong that I had no choice but to follow it and see where it would lead me. That was when I moved to Northern California to live with my dad and eventually join the Jesuit Volunteer Corp. I worked one year as an activity coordinator for four senior citizen centers in Juneau, Alaska. I met my husband of 18 years three weeks before the end of that year. We married and had three beautiful children. My healing career began shortly after my babies were born.

~ My Beginning ~

As a child, many experiences lifted me into recognition of the path that was before me. I had what some people might call a *sacred contract* with my brother Danny at six months old. My mother and siblings offered him the greatest of love, yet Danny became physically worse in time due to a heart that was much larger than his little body could handle. He was one of the first heart patients in Los Angeles at that age ever to have been operated on. Unfortunately, he did not make it.

Fortunately, it brought me into awareness, and I became alive with pure knowledge at six months old. I woke up to the spirit I am without age, without attachments, and physically and consciously became aware that I was back in a body. Looking and gazing at my hands, my inner voice was saying, "These will do." As I looked at the dresser, the curtains, the window, etc. I realized that I would need to remember this in order to eventually tell others, and mostly, my mother. The vivid memory of my grandmother coming into the room at that time and changing my diaper is as fresh within me now as it was 53 years ago. This is a direct memory of this waking up process to where I am today.

At six years old, I was sitting in my front yard playing with a blade of grass. I remember examining little hairs on this blade and asking myself how a tiny blade of grass could grow hair. Suddenly, my eyes went blind for approximately two minutes with bright white light. The neighborhood was missing from my vision. For a second, it crossed my mind that we might have been bombed, as Los Angeles was having air raids in the early 60's, yet there was *peace* inside of me.

I found out many years later that this was a *light experience* understood by mystics as an initiation into the world of mysticism. My memory from this moment forward would be sharp and aware as an observer. The schools I attended, the animals we had, et al would be in the forefront of my mind, yet I would only refer to these times if there were a reason to. I spoke to dogs and cats telepathically, and I knew they could hear me. They actually spoke back, and the language they exuded was my language.

I used to walk to school with my sister and a friend every morning. I attended a Catholic school and wore a uniform. One day when I was in second grade, my mom had changed detergents when washing this uniform. The new detergent had me itching so badly that I lost consciousness during class. Instead of falling over, I transcended out of my body similar to a near death experience; however, I went into a trance-type state. I remember the teacher calling my name, and my continuous stare out the window was soon interrupted. Back to my body I went.

The tingling was too much as this reaction was profound. One thing it taught me was that I could transcend during any situation yet stay remotely conscious enough to grasp what was happening at the time. This was the beginning of seeing my life as a mystic, or better yet, an observer. The best part was I learned that I didn't have to attach to any outcome. Instead I could be larger in my spirit and still be aware.

Eventually, being present and focused became more magnified with the ability to transcend when necessary. I truly believe that within me, becoming the healer I am today was fed by this action. Mainly, I could see differently from others' perspectives without attachment. As I got older, I was quietly aware of true friendships. I watched certain people in my classes and discovered who was real and who wasn't. Somehow even at a young age, this seemed very important.

I find childhood incredibly important for everyone because it's in these informative years that we make our minds up as to how we will be and what behaviors we take on when we get older. Now that we are in the time of changes in 2012, I find most people have blockages in this area that are in the way of their spiritual growth. Mostly the age of six is when we determine our behavior through the decisions we make for survival.

My passion, as I share this information with you, is to accomplish recognition from our childhood to where we are now. There has never been a better time to achieve everything we ever dreamed, to see our past and acknowledge it as just that and to realize that a new life means you discover yourself as a divine human ready to see life as an absolute adventure with Spirit, your ancestors, your guides, and the awareness that we are never alone. The acknowledgements I've carried are what excite me about sharing all of the truths I have found in humanity as each day brings in further growth for all of us to be a part of, to create with, and have each other to lean on.

My clients have shown me huge parts of a global understanding as they have taught me not only to see from a healer's insightful recognition but also to listen beyond my own ears. This is what I feel has made me the healer I am today. What each person offers as they agreed to come in for their healings is making our learning more productive in this field of healing…not only in my office, but for the world.

I appreciate each one of you who are reading this book, and I hope these insights of lessons learned and knowledge gained open doors for you. It gives me great pleasure to bring a different perspective with great understandings to the light of recognition for each of you, and more importantly, for our world to hear in this time of change.

Blessings, Mona~

1.

CONSCIOUS HEALTH IN A CHANGING WORLD

"Doctors don't know everything! They understand matter, not spirit. You and I live in spirit."
- William Saroyan, The Human Comedy

We are in a changing world where awareness is beginning to lead humanity into more creative and responsible health. As individuals waking up to the dilemma in our health care systems, we recognize the need for change and realize that these times are highly significant for all of us. It's time to come together in unity and help each other to heal.

For thirty years I have seen people search for answers to many of their questions regarding health in general. Fortunately, in my work as a Medical Intuitive Energy Runner, I have been able to tap into the most important lessons a client is going through. This is cellular memory in action. When a repeated experience comes to the surface (We call it a "pattern."), then we are able to identify it and come to grips with it.

Our ultimate goal is to discover for ourselves a place inside where there is contentment, satisfaction, and peace. It is a place of surrender, yet empowerment. Most people are still searching, as day to day stresses are getting the best of us.

Unfortunately, as this happens, our immune systems break down as our nervous systems get maxed. The adrenal glands become tired due to the constant thought processes, and the "fight or flight" response kicks in. Sleep is interrupted, and clear thinking can feel like a thing of the past. We tend to use up our energy on patterns associated with daily routines that are about how we think we are surviving or handling the demands of the day.

For years, enlightened authors and positive speakers have spoken of meditation. Yet, if in our world, we do not seem to be able to find enough time to even sit down and eat, let alone meditate, how will we ever become healthy and stay that way?

~ Let Truth Be Known ~

What we call "health care" today is actually an oxymoron. Simply put, I have yet to find health in this massive corporation where drugs rule, surgeries are at times unnecessary, diagnoses are out of line, doctors are busy with too many demands, costs are relentlessly criminal, insurance companies are denying claims, and last of all, our own lives have now been given over to someone who has no idea who we are.

On many levels, we know that this way of thinking about our health has been accepted and demanded for way too long. There are good doctors with very good hearts who generally would love to see a patient heal. However, even the best of doctors know that we are ultimately responsible for taking care of ourselves since they and their families also get sick and have to find answers. This is the way of life. Answers to illness are not found in prescription drugs. Most drugs stop your brain from associating what pain is and why it's there in the first place. Working with pain is doable with different forms of treatment; but when we drug ourselves, we obviously become dependent once again.

In all the years I've worked in health care, I've seen that we have chosen to be submissive to others' ideas so as not to take responsibility for our own health. Then we can even blame someone else if something should go wrong with the medicines we are taking! Take note of that word: "Medicine."

~ Unrealistic Medication ~

A Medicine Cabinet Life

One day I went to the spa downstairs from my office to soak in the hot tub after a long day of seeing clients. Suddenly I heard a woman's voice asking me if I were the Massage Therapist upstairs. I said, "Yes," wondering if she were going to ask for an appointment. Much to my surprise, she asked if she could talk to me privately in the sauna. She told me that she was on Prozac for six years. Her doctor kept her on it because it helped her depression. After about five years, she began to lose her memory. Soon after that, she was having trouble with her speech. Between her forgetfulness and then her slurred speech, she was sent to another doctor to be checked out with tests. The doctors had diagnosed her with Alzheimer's disease and were ready to prescribe more drugs.

Fortunately, her daughter was very aware that her mother was not one that she would have pegged for getting Alzheimer's. She insisted on her seeing an acupuncturist for her condition. The acupuncturist recommended that she go back to her original doctor and have her tapered off of Prozac, which her daughter then did. The agreeable doctor concurred, and within a few weeks, this woman was speaking normally. After a few months, she was steadily getting better. She wanted to tell me about it so that I could, in turn, tell my clients about the dangers of Prozac. This woman was in fine condition at the age of 62. This happened in the year 1992.

Statistics are something I take with a grain of salt. The same goes for medical studies. These studies change from one day to another, and there are thousands of people who are not included in statistics. No one can ever really know the truth of these tests; however, it isn't rocket science when we see the amount of prescription overuse in today's treatments. I read recently that prescription drugs, taken as directed, have killed over 200,000 people a year. I watched a program on television that stated that there are over 200 pill mills in Florida alone! These places dish out oxycodone, and people fly there to pick it up to sell it later.

People are addicted, and people are dying. In truth, people are scared. They are ultimately lost and do not know where to turn. Some of the ones interviewed claimed they are needy for money and are in pain on many levels. We *do not* know all of the reasons for this crime being acceptable in our country alone. We *do* know that there are other cures, other options, and other places for people to seek help.

In this book, it is my passion to share what I have learned over many years. I have worked at a rate that most people would have a difficult time keeping up with, yet my passion for the work I have done and conditions I have seen have led me to where I am today with the same passion I had when I began this work.

In 1998, I made an appointment with a doctor who was in charge of several clinics in the Mid-West. His family lived in my town, and the wife and I were friends. I happened to be at their home one evening after telling his wife that I would love to talk to him. I had so much to share and didn't know what to do with all of this information that felt like it wanted to explode out of me. I found out that evening that he was a part of the National Institute of Health (NIH), making it even better for me since I was aware that Deepak Chopra was also a part of NIH.

I went on to explain to this doctor that I had the ability, or "gift" as some call it, to know *why* a person comes down with an illness…no matter what it was. I told him that in order to get any form of illness or disease, you have to have a resonating factor somewhere inside you that makes you vulnerable to that condition in the first place. Hereditary information is a definite possibility; however, if people understood that we are *not* our parents and have a different soul altogether, we wouldn't have to have any form of sickness, or even a heart attack, et al. We could be conscious of viewing life from our own eyes rather than someone else's.

I figured since there was a part of National Institute of Health called "Alternative and Complementary Medicine," this doctor might see the importance of what I was sharing and help me to find a way to teach them what I knew. These researchers could have a gold mine of information, respectively with understanding personality traits, etc. that cause illness in the first place. This information I had could help guide them into more knowledge for the sake of healing and quantum facts.

Unfortunately, the doctor looked at me strangely and proceeded to ask me why I had come to him. He wanted to know if I were looking for a grant. About that time, I began to feel as though no one would hear me. Bottled up inside me was a medicine cabinet of knowledge, and he wanted to know if a grant is what I wanted!

Saddened and disappointed, I made the decision to keep working as usual on clients and learn even more so that one day I could share it with the world. Well, today is that day. The timing is crucial and appropriate now, as more and more writers and speakers are addressing the need to change this system we call "health care."

In the last year, I have been acknowledged by many people, as my information has been getting out with the articles on my website, etc. I recently have been on five radio shows with great responses. More importantly, with one radio program, I was asked by the host how I saw the future of health care. My answer was, "By healing each other, of course!" The radio host denied that this could work, and actually thought it would be humorous to make fun of me. He indicated that our country would never go for this and would never allow the *powers to be* to stand down for any reason. He commented that the world would never accept that simple concept. Again my response was, "Never say 'Never.'"

If more people understood that we are all energy and that pain is energy, they might understand that we make our own choices when it comes to our health. The only difficulty is that most people don't have a role model who understands the concepts of living that free us and lead us to real health. Health has to be considered as the whole unit.

In the next few chapters, I will discuss these sacred concepts and truths for these changes to be understood and acknowledged. My Cherokee mentor of 12 years used to say, "All it takes is the desire to know and the desire to act in order to heal." I found this to be very true. Yet also, if we take the word *responsibility*, we will see that it's not a word that we have to fear. Many people fear what they see as responsibility because they feel as though they aren't good enough and might fail in a task, even in their own healing. Responsibility alone will change our lives and the lives of others. The healing within us, once it is understood, will generate energy around you where others will sense you are healthy, and they too will want some of that energy!

~ Energy Transference ~

I remember in 1993 when Deepak Chopra came out with one of the most profound books I have ever read. *Ageless Body, Timeless Mind* gave us a clear look at what this energy was all about. In the book he talks about different studies that were done in laboratories with rats. One study shows two cages, each containing the same amount of rats. One cage of rats was given love. They were petted and talked to each day for weeks. The other cage of rats was left alone except to be fed. After about three weeks, both cages were given poison with their food. The rats that were left alone died. The rats that were given love and petted lived as though they were fed the same food as usual. With those rats, it was the transference of love that kept them alive.

We all know that alternative therapies are getting more popular by the day. It is now common for people to receive chiropractic work as well as acupuncture, massage, Reiki, and even flower essences (all of which are vibrational healing therapies). There are clinics for amino acid therapy and many body, mind, spirit clinics for getting a whole body adjustment. All of these therapies have something in common. Unlike the medical profession, they all have an understanding of energy and even more importantly, energy transference.

When I was in nursing, I was in a patient's room, and she asked me why I was a nurse in neurology. I told her I loved the work and enjoyed meeting people; it made my day go more quickly. I also mentioned that I had just finished massage school and received my license. (Having received my massage license, the excitement was almost overwhelming because I had worked to pass that test to the absolute best of my ability. And man, what a test! If you haven't taken a massage therapy course, you would never have an idea of how difficult it really is. You really need to know your muscles, insertions, counter muscle, et al.)

She smiled and said, "I own a diet center, and I would love it if you would come and work there doing massage. I could get you all the clients you would need." I have to admit that I was tempted by the offer. Telling my husband at the time was going to be a bigger challenge than taking the position! Needless to say, I accepted her offer and started my massage practice in 1990. I quit my nursing job to do this full time, and you can imagine knowing you were ready now to follow your passion. Oh boy!

I started out renting a small space behind the diet center. The excitement was almost overwhelming because I knew this was it! I even had quit my nursing job, without telling my husband at first, because I was SO ready to help others the way I saw healing could be… absolutely personal!

Then my first client scheduled through the diet center. I was all gussied up and ready to do my job when I was taken by a huge surprise. She was suicidal! She weighed 300 pounds, and she was upset yet acted strong. Her anger of being overweight and "not good enough" had really made that Goddess part of her turn to despair. Her frustration about her life, her weight, and her brother taking charge in a family business had made her jealous and angry.

She shared with me the upsets and frustrations as I was working on her body. So I gave her a Mona massage and consoled her through the only wisdom I had to offer at that time. After the session was finished, she said a polite thank you, and we parted ways.

Little did I know that as we were in this space, I was taking on her pain. It wasn't so much physical; it was mostly emotional. Needless to say, when I was done with the session, I began to feel sick to my stomach and very dizzy. Fortunately, I had no other clients and decided to go home. At first I thought I was getting sick. But how could something come on so fast when I was fine an hour before? As I was trying to cook dinner for my family, I became clammy, and my emotions were heading through the roof.

That night, I threw up several times. I also had the feeling that I wasn't "me" anymore. I felt angry, strong, and now I was really feeling sick. I curled up in a fetal position and went under the kitchen table and rocked back and forth. It was very disturbing not to be able to gather myself. Most importantly, I remember feeling that maybe I would become insane and not come out of it. What would happen to my kids? I felt crazy. My husband was thinking about calling someone for help. I told him to leave me alone. He helped me go to bed. (Fortunately, he didn't call the men in the white coats.) That night I cried myself to sleep.

I woke up in the morning feeling just fine. No hangover from the energy of that woman. No problems at all! My emotions were intact, and I felt good. Maybe I'd be ok? Whew! What a relief! I realized I had put my family in a" tizzy" the night before, not knowing what was wrong with me.

The rest of that week was good. Then I heard from the diet center that the woman who was my first client had made another appointment! I started thinking, "YIKES! How can I tell them that I don't want to see her? Do I cancel? Do I tell her she needs to see someone else? Would it crush her if I told her that I don't want to see her?" Well, after the initial scream from the inside, I calmed down and told myself that if I got through this one, I could do it again (maybe). Rather than being a coward, I did it. I bit the bullet and decided to give it another shot.

The day came, and she walked in for her session. WOW! She was wearing a red dress, and she was beautiful. Her hair was gorgeous, her make-up was pristine, and she had lost five pounds in a week! I almost gasped as I wanted to say, "What happened to you?" Instead I asked her how she felt and told her she looked stunning.

She said she was happily grateful for the work we had done the week before. She told me that she didn't know what

I had done, but whatever it was, she was a new lady. Boy, did it show! What just happened? When I massaged her, she felt better, more peaceful, and she even laughed at one of my silly jokes! She then gave me a huge hug and said she'd never felt better! Good! I really didn't want to tell her I felt like absolute "you know what" that first night!

The truth is that lesson was for me. Once I was able to get through the initial chaos of transference, I could go about realizing that maybe this was normal. Perhaps everyone who does healing work feels this? Anyone who does any healing work, no matter where you come from, race, religion, et al, feels the person they care about, one way or another. This is truly natural for everyone, but maybe not at the level I ran into from the start! (Thank God, or we'd be in a world of hurt!) Transference is strictly the combined energy of the knowledge that we all are *one*. It's osmosis in action.

This experience was when I first realized that this is something that people wouldn't get in a hospital or even in a counselor's office. I actually felt honored. From then on, the transference became easier. I realized that as soon as I recognized that these strange feelings were foreign and not a part of *my* world, they had to be someone else's. This, then, became my new way of healing and helping others. I wasn't afraid of transference after that, even though it seemed I could have had a reason to be. I trusted that this was God's way of interconnecting all of us. We are all energy and we can pick up on people around us and even those in other places.

It's like using a cell phone. We have connection when we are dialed in, but we can hang up anytime we choose. We wouldn't hang up on anyone during a conversation for the most part, so why would we ignore a client or a loved one in their moment of need? We are transducers. We are givers (transmitters) and receivers of light, love, information, and communication. When a student would come in and tell me that transference really bothered them and that they were too sensitive, I warned them about being in this profession and told them they might do better taking a nine-to-five job for now. However, they would still be sensitive and would still pick up on co-workers and family members, etc. It would be better to learn the lessons of self-recognition now for tools to have in their future.

I taught classes soon after and showed massage therapists how to overlap the transference effect and *still* feel normal after a long day's work. To be a very good healer, you feel the pain, the emotion, the hardness, the insecurity of the person you are treating. Buying it as ours only attaches us to that sensation, and that's what is overwhelming. If it isn't ours, we need to *feel* that so as to help the person we love or care for. We can still be individual and even stronger in the long run when we aren't afraid of listening with our own body. This alone is a healing. Actually, this type of transference happens all the time for us, whether we're aware of it or not. We better get used to this occurrence because the future will prove this to intensify.

We are being magnetized as the shift gets stronger in our solar system. It is also happening in our physical system.

We are seeing more people getting illnesses that are unrecognized by our physicians. More conditions in the body are occurring to which doctors might say, "It's all in your head," especially if they can't find anything wrong. You can have low back pain and go in for an x-ray, only to find everything appears normal. At this point, due to our insensitive nature, does anyone even know that you hurt?

Many conditions today will be due to a high voltage of frequencies that are lifting your old patterns and emotions out of the body. The cells are actually *crying out* for healing and for freedom! The increases of solar flares from the Sun are proving that our bodies are being affected as we let go of old patterns. These patterns have to come to the surface to express themselves after being hidden within us for so long. In other words, these flares seem to be raising our consciousness and awareness while confusing and overwhelming us at the same time. As the movie line says, "Something's gotta give." This is why the build up of emotions seems to be creating havoc in sensitive people.

However, we are actually becoming like metal filings or fragments being pulled into the light. In order to do this, we must be cleared out of 3rd Dimensional thinking and living. This clearing ultimately will be our best friend. The love of the Universe moves us into a new realm called Unity Consciousness: Unity eventually in our cells, in our lives, and in our world.

I am not religious by nature; I am Spiritual and encompass all races, creeds, and religions. However, a quote in the Bible has stayed with me for many years. When Jesus said, "Where two or more are gathered," I pondered this as a child. I knew many adults who were confused by it or brushed it off with their limited understandings and taught just that. Jesus, in my opinion, didn't mean anything light-hearted or airy-fairy. Every time he spoke, there was a tornado of information and meaning behind his words. So, "Where two or more are gathered" became the most important message this teacher ever offered.

In healing, one person reads and recognizes what someone else is experiencing. Once this conversation, whether it is aloud or silent, is acknowledged, it becomes recognition of energy. Therefore, the releases from any form of communication happen automatically and can be healed, and new adventures are developed. This is what I call the "big bang." It is like an explosion of releases within us when we discover the "A-HA" moment…or a resonance of the truth within us. There are a million big bangs every day. So when two or more are gathered, "two" can include anything, not just people. This is extremely important for the future of health care. We don't have to have a Master's degree in healing or in science. We just need the comprehension and the compassion for true healing to occur.

~ Beyond Limitation ~

It has been reported in medical studies that the phenomenon of energy transference in hospitals, nursing homes, etc. has made an impact in our world. One story was of a woman named Claire Sylvia who was in need of a heart transplant. She was in the hospital, very weak and dying. The doctors had not yet found a heart for her and were still looking. Time was very short. Much to their surprise, there was a phone call stating that an accident had just occurred, and a man on a motorcycle had been killed. He was a donor, so they immediately set her up for surgery and performed the transplant.

Upon awakening, the nurses asked Claire if they could get her anything, and her response shocked everyone when she said, "Yes, I would like a beer and French fries." The man who had died just hours before this transplant had been on his motorcycle at McDonald's getting French fries when he was hit by a car. Not only was her response amazing but so was the fact that she never drank beer! Later she had written a book called *A Change Of Heart*. (That book was also forwarded by Bernie Siegel, M.D.)

This happened in my practice throughout the years as well. I had a client who had just lost her son to a motor vehicle accident. He was nineteen years old and loved to fly fish, drive his truck, and be with friends. He wanted to have a family and children some day. His mother loved him so very much and decided to donate his organs when the time came for someone in need. Well, that time came. Her son's kidneys were given to a man who had been on dialysis for a while. When it came to his needing kidneys, he received them from the nineteen- year-old's donation.

A year later, my client received a letter from the man with her son's kidneys. He did not know this family or anything about what had happened. However, he did find out where to send this letter. Upon her visit to see me one wonderful day, she showed me the letter stating that the recipient of her son's kidneys felt like a twenty-year-old kid.

He said he began fly fishing and felt surges of energy to be with his four children again. His gratitude was overwhelming, and he had to find where to send this letter. My client and I were both crying as she was reading it. I felt that this beautiful connection was occurring right in front of us, and we were both so blessed to be able to share this with each other.

It was then that I *knew* that there were no boundaries whatsoever to energy healing. Quantum awareness would take place even faster now as my recognition to all healing was opened wider to all possibilities. I turned on the hose, if you will, and from that moment, I challenged any form of healing to become greater and more productive. I knew my healing work was strong. Now it was about to become stronger. Realizing that since this was so real and mind blowing, then what about other transplants and blood transfusions? I have seen it, felt it, and even healed it with clients.

When we or someone we know receives a blood transfusion or any kind of transplant, it is clear that the recipient takes on the energies of the person donating. This is new to us, but since we have the recognition now, we can also understand that our intent for any transplant makes a difference when we see this donated organ or blood as a clean and purified living part in us or our loved one. We only need to put our focus and intent into the new part coming into the body. Instead of just having the surgery, transplant, or blood transfusion, we are more than capable of energetically changing any unpurified part to being purified along with trusting that all will go well. Just as Dr. Masaru Emoto wrote in his book *Water Crystal Healing*, we can heal ourselves through music, words, and a combination of images.

~ Natural Wisdom ~

The future of health care will have to be known as "living simply so others can simply live." Eventually we will not have a medical profession to run to every time we get a runny nose. We will not always have insurance companies to pay our bills for us, and we will not have accurate diagnoses to depend on for taking a prescribed medication.

As a global community, we have become unconsciously lazy in our own care; however, times are changing quickly. People ARE waking up to seeing this. We are living more from the heart as we feel more with compassion. Our children are hearing and learning these concepts, and there are many parents who are listening as well. We are ultimately tired of the game. I see many people who are asking questions and taking back their power. They just need direction.

Honesty is the best policy. To truly heal from our patterns and our individual hurts and pains, by acknowledging where or how they got there, we can counteract the condition. We can even go back in time and train our minds to overcome the very things that hurt us in the first place. Hypnosis works for many people with this very same concept. We do not need to depend on hypnosis, either. Even hypnosis doesn't work for everyone because some have a sense of wanting to be in control and do it themselves. If that's the case, more power to them!

We are coming into Oneness as we DO have each other. Our ancients and Shamans who lived in tribes (and still do) represent natural healing. Not only do they know the power of this oneness, but also they respect it and live their entire lives by it. This is happening in the Oneness today. Soon we will begin to feel lighter as time continues to magnify us into higher realms on our planet. The future of health care is going to have to be simplified. Herbs we grow will be understood through the feeling nature of what they are saying to the body. We can interpret these energies just as much as when we read someone's energy field. Flowers will be for color therapy and as essences to take internally.

We will have to learn to listen, to slow down, and to still our minds from the need for gratification. Remembering that health comes from knowledge and acceptance, we as a community of people will realize that we are all healers by nature. We are all empaths to some degree, meaning empathetic transducers. We have all been given the gifts of caring and, of course, love.

Once we understand this sacred language that our bodies provide, we too will be magnifying ourselves back into a world of grace, beauty, and, ultimately teamwork of healing together. This is how we can respectfully give back to the Universe what the Universe is giving to us. This, my dear friends, is how we live in and with Nature. It's a whole language of adapting to who and what we really are.

2.

RECONSTRUCTING HUMAN AWARENESS

*"Align each decision you make with the person you want to be.
If you do, you'll always know what action will create
what you want." - Nick Bogatin*

Many years ago, I saw an interview with the legendary American scholar, Joseph Campbell. Joseph was a man who understood the patterns in human behavior as he explained it to us through myths and storytelling. I was, needless to say, glued to the television at a young age as I watched him come alive with passion in the Bill Moyer's series, *The Power of Myth*.

I wanted so badly to remember his words, his teaching, and his humor. I knew I could go back and buy the tape, but I chose to embody his wisdom. His teachings became the truth of my life, and I knew it. Back in the days of the late 70's and early 80's, few people (compared to today) understood these teachings.

He wrote a book called *The Hero with a Thousand Faces* in which he tells the story of *"The Hero's Journey."* It describes the typical adventure of the archetype known as the Hero, the person who goes out and achieves great deeds on behalf of the group or the tribe. Campbell explores the theory that important myths from around the world which have survived for thousands of years all share a fundamental structure called a "mono-myth."

The mono-myth of the summary of his book is this: *"A hero ventures forth from the world of common day into a region of supernatural wonder. Fabulous forces are there encountered and a decisive victory is won. The hero comes back from this mysterious adventure with the power to bestow boons on his fellow man."*

The number of stages and the summary of the steps are as follows:

"The Ordinary World"

Here, the hero is uneasy and basically unaware; however, this is the one introduced so that the audience can identify with his situation. The hero is being torn, and a type of polarity is pulling him in different directions, causing a dilemma. This person does not know his potential or calling.

"The Call to Adventure"

From something rising up inside this person, his situation gets shaken. Pressure comes, and the hero must face the beginnings of the change.

"Refusal of the Call"

This is known as "the reluctant hero." Fear of the unknown sets in and he tries to run from the adventure, however briefly. In concordance to this emotion, a sense of duty, obligation, or even insecurity can bring in inadequacy. The hero wonders if there's danger ahead.

"Meeting with the Mentor"

Once the hero commits to the quest, he finds the teacher. A guide appears as a helper or even an ordinary man, who helps him on the journey to courage and wisdom.

"Crossing the Threshold"

The end of Act One demonstrates that this is the point where the hero crosses into the field of adventure and leaves the Ordinary World. He becomes better adapted to unfamiliar values.

"Tests, Allies, and Enemies"

These are what the hero must undergo in order to begin this transformation. A new approach, the confrontation with death, and in a single moment, the greatest fear is faced, and out from death comes a new life.

"The Reward"

Treasures are won by facing death; however, danger still lurks as there could still be a belief that the treasure may become lost.

"The Road Back"

As the story is almost finished, the hero is driven to complete the adventure. He needs to revisit the mentor to learn new mentoring. Then he returns to the path he started on...reborn.

"The Resurrection"

The hero becomes tested again as he ventures on the threshold of home. By the hero's actions, after he encounters another brush with death, he becomes purified and reaches higher levels, proving the lessons were learned.

"Return With Elixir"

The hero now returns home and achieves the goal of the quest. This elixir is not a plant or a medicine as we know it. It is the balance between the material and the spiritual world. Now there is freedom from fear and from fear of death. The hero is transformed.

As you can see by the story itself, this may sound very familiar to you. For those of you who resonate to it, you can see that this is ALL of our paths that we are on today. We are, by right, our very own heroes writing our very own books.

~ It Begins with Awareness ~

When we think about "how" to begin to shift our thoughts, it must come first through a circumstance's occurring and then being brought to our awareness for a reason. Awareness truly comes from the heart through emotions. Here are some ways to help you identify how awareness occurs:

1) A reaction we are having to a current situation

2) A frustration because we are not able to control an outcome

3) A very happy and enlightening moment with a Friend and then an awakening as to why we just became "happy"

4) A dream that encourages us to "feel" connected, whether we remember the whole thing or not

5) Hearing a song on the radio that triggers a memory of someone or a time in your life

I could go on about how awareness happens. However, the bottom line is that as we get our "A-HA" moment, it is important to acknowledge it! Since each of us has a different concept of what is important to our own growth, we can develop into our Self and allow these encouraging "A-HA" moments to take a priority in our consciousness.

If we live more in the moment, we can live in continual recognition of how we make decisions and react appropriately in the moment. We will find that our "A-HA" moments become more frequent. As a result, life begins to feel lighter. Your body feels lighter. You aren't as tired. Energy turns into vitality because you are being fed. So we can ask ourselves the question, "How can I achieve these 'A-HA' moments faster?"

The answer to that question has to do with insecurities due to old fears. If we had no fears from prior experiences (not just from this one lifetime), we wouldn't have any reason to "hold back." Our knowledge would be happening at such a great rate! We would have absolutely *nothing* stopping us from being everything we choose to be and become in our world today.

Obviously, insecurities have been a part of life for eons! Fears are there on very subconscious levels for protection. But protection of what? Have we actually detached ourselves to believe we were enhancing our Selves when really it's been fear all along?

So many people have believed they were doing the "right" thing in life for themselves through an action, and then they found later that somehow things didn't turn out the way they'd hoped. Why? They attracted an outcome through a level of fear without recognition. Many people would say, "It was God's plan." Or they would believe that it just was not that important, and life took a course because they weren't good enough.

It's amazing how we see ourselves and judge due to an outcome, but that's our human limitation. If we have the ability to do anything, feel anything, and see in any way we want to, then what could possibly be stopping this amazing concept called "Sacred Sight"?

~ Sacred Sight ~

I looked in the dictionary recently to see how many definitions I could find under the word "sacred." There must have been over 30 definitions, not to mention the Bible quotes! One, for example, is the "Sacred Heart of Jesus." *Sacred*, in this case, is more of an adjective describing the purity of heart seen by many about Jesus. Just as this meaning arises, other definitions, such as "divine" or even "holy," come up. I see this word as a reason to call something "respectable." A *true respect* for the human body is how I revere it as sacred. So what would the idea of sacred sight mean?

When we look at a rock, we realize that this rock has been here for eons. It became a rock simply through its own evolution. We might decide to use the phrase, "If this rock could talk..." By using a phrase like this one, we could say that we SAW this rock as sacred. In other words, we are paying attention to the fact that we respect this rock and the years it has seen instead of taking it for granted and not giving it any thought at all. This is what is known as Sacred Sight. When you are respectful to others, to any circumstance or situation, then in truth, you hold this awareness as sacred. You are the Observer and are not interfering in their process. You see with your heart. This is how we begin to understand the concept of Sacred Sight.

Once we begin to allow ourselves to get to this awareness, we then can go deeper with the feelings of being connected to all things! Native American tradition has taught this for thousands of years. Where did this ability within all of us get so caught up in separation? Being *one* with all things requires us to simply know that we are one with all things. It's simple because it's true.

Many of us have seen ourselves separate from the Earth, the Ocean, and Nature. Some of us have done so out of what we've considered respect or awe. It's wonderful to know the "gratitude of the magnitude;" however, power is *within* all. When we truly connect to our surroundings, we feel a sense of peace. I'm talking about feeling nature and its magnificence *within* ourselves. When we connect ourselves, then we become that same magnitude within, which holds the balance of expansiveness, completion, clarity, and divine purpose.

~ Hereditary Gifts from Earth ~

"Whatever does not exist in the body can't be found in the Universe. Whatever exists in the Universe can be found in the body." – Ghandi

In Gregg Braden's You Tube presentation on Consciousness, he describes how the magnetic fields of the Earth have been proven to be affected by events, such as 9/11, only 15 minutes after the first plane hit the World Trade Center. Science has clearly documented these conditions of the human heart to reflect the spikes in these magnetic fields through satellite activity. Simply from our emotions! When we tune in to our heart's electromagnetic emotions, the Earth can hear us and aligns to this as well. If everyone had only anger and pain, the Earth would HAVE to act the same in order for us to see the mirror as a whole. It may be that we have to feel shaken to awaken, or maybe we'll learn to advance from clarity this time. (Jesus would be so proud!)

So if this is really the case of connection, we must be more cognizant of our responsibility within our Selves *and* within the entire world. What a wonderful responsibility to have at a time most necessary in our world! What a feeling to know you and I are contributing to this magnificent purpose! We've waited for years for others to come forward and have cursed that which doesn't relate to our idea of love or what we felt justified in. Why not become the example we want others to see, feel within ourselves, and get simplified? Again, it can be so simple.

There is a wonderful slide show that's been going around the internet since 1998. I just received it a few days ago, just in time to get it in the book! It clearly is a wonderful piece of information about certain fruits and vegetables that resemble parts of our body. For example, when you slice a carrot, did you know that it looks like an eye with the iris and a pupil? Of course, carrots have Vitamin A that is good for the eyes!

The list continues....

Tomatoes: There are four chambers when you slice a tomato. The heart has four chambers. They are both red. Tomatoes have lycopine, which feeds the heart and the blood.

Grapes: In the bunch, they resemble the shape of the heart. Alone they resemble a cell. Grapes are known as anti-bacteria cleansers in the body and are good for certain cancers.

Walnuts: These actually look like brains! They have a wrinkled appearance, and it looks like they include cerebrums and cerebellums. Walnuts help develop more than three dozen neurotransmitters for brain function. They even have a fold. Creepy or not, it's true!

Kidney beans: Yes, they look like kidneys. They even help maintain kidney function.

Celery, Bok Choy, Rhubarb: They all resemble the bones. These veggies actually improve bone strength. Bones are 23% sodium; these are 23% sodium. The skeletal system needs sodium to keep the marrow strong.

Avocados: These actually take nine months to grow and ripen. Can you guess what they look like and what they're for? Avocados balance female hormones and look like a woman's cervix. They've been known to help prevent cervical cancer.

Pears and Eggplants: These are similar to the avocado, but they look more like a womb. Their nutritional benefit is also important.

Figs: These hang by two's. Believe it or not, they've been known for helping increase sperm count in men and helping them to overcome sterility!

Sweet Potatoes: Okay, this one looks like a pancreas, and it helps to balance glycemic conditions related to diabetes.

Olives: Olives help with function and health of the ovaries. Well, they kind of resemble them, too.

Oranges , Grapefruits, and Citrus: These maintain the movement of lymph to and from the breasts. They also resemble the mammary glands!

Onions: These are like the body's cells. Eating onions actually helps the body in the way that an antibiotic does. They clean waste from a cell. Onions also produce tears, which wash the tissue around the eye. Its cousin, garlic, has very similar effects on the body's immune system.

Of course, these are to name only a few. How fascinating it is when we pay attention. I don't know about you, but it makes me love our Earth Mother more all the time.

No matter what part of the world you are from, for thousands of years, herbs have been known to heal the body. There are 4,000 herbs in America being used to cure conditions in our systems, and that's only the "known" ones. I have never picked up or held a plant without it telling me what it does. It relates through the same means as the body. It gives your body its language for you, just by holding it in your left hand and by your feeling the sensation. Since this is our receiver side, there is nothing we can't determine as "good for us" just by holding it directly and getting the result in your body.

If we can connect this strongly with osmosis of other life forms, just think of all the things we could be missing out on. What about the animal kingdom? We have heard of having a totem animal. How is it we can relate so well to a cougar, an elk, a rabbit, etc. and then not get the sense that all things are connected? Again, another reason to acknowledge how we can change our world by working together and considering health care from the heart. We sure have waited for it! I'd say for over 2,000 years!

Our part in this world is exceptionally and integrally important, and what we do with it makes a difference. How you live it day by day and what you do with it is totally up to you. The "drop in the water" effect is happening second by second. Our words, our thoughts, our perceptions, and our actions are all changing this world, seconds at a time.

~ Energy Transference Happens: How Do We Know? ~

As I know how important it is to read the body, I can tell you that healers with this capability are profound in the here and now and for our future in the profession of healing. So often students have asked me how they would know whether how they felt after being around someone (talking to them or working on them) belonged to them or the other person.

There are different answers to this question.
1) Did you feel this way before you had the encounter?
2) Is the way you're feeling related to a mood that you go through on a regular basis?
3) Does it feel foreign?
4) Do you hurt in a place you didn't hurt before you had this encounter?

These are some of the ways you can identify if this is transference. Simply put, recognize it could be someone else's pain, emotion, or even their thoughts. Take the guilt off yourself.

Transference happens in our own homes. When our kids are sick, we take on their illness so they don't have to suffer. Most parents don't even know this happens! Or the child will take yours so you don't have to experience it. (Here we thought it was just contagious!) Have you ever been around anyone with head lice for just a moment and then started itching? That's an obvious example; however, take that to larger levels, and you'll find there's much more we don't realize. The thoughts of your friends or partner can influence your very own thought process and turn you into who they are rather than who you are in any given situation. This is no different then when we see our high school kids perform under peer pressure. We as adults usually don't see it for ourselves.

Another interesting point when it comes to health is related to parents. When we were growing up in our parents' home, we didn't know that, for the most part, we wanted to be pleasing and accepted. Most of us didn't understand why we didn't meet the grade with our moms or our dads. (This is why counselors ask you, "Did you get along with your mom?")

Typically, we eventually take on the behavior of our parents in one way or another without realizing it. This, too, is natural. Dr. Bruce Lipton, author of *Biology Beyond Belief* and most recently, *Spontaneous Evolution*, talks about the environment's being our difficulty relating to clarity within ourselves. That includes the subconscious belief systems we carry within us that do not actually belong to us. Maybe it was our father's belief that we had to work hard to make a living. Therefore, if we lose our job, we feel as though we have failed and cannot see that we possibly will be given a new position to use our talents differently. This is what our home environment was like.

We chose, on some level, to buy into the concepts of our families and our peers, not taking full responsibility for our own truth. In our world today, it's important to ask yourself if the feelings you feel and the way you react is yours... or theirs.

The reason I bring this up is that when it comes to our health, we ALWAYS have choices in our responses, our actions, and our reactions. (Life would be so boring, actually, if we were clones!) Doctors tell us that when we enter their office, we must fill out a form about ourselves. The first question is usually, "Are your mother and father still alive?" Then, "Does anybody in your family have heart problems?" This list goes on so the doctor can get to know your bloodline history.

~ Bloodline "Hand-Me-Downs?" ~

When we talk about patterns in the body, we need to understand that these are changeable. If they weren't, we might as well curl up and tell ourselves that we are doomed and life isn't worth living!! Ugh.

In the medical profession, we have understood that disease can come from hereditary bloodlines. When they talk about heart disease, MS, diabetes, or even cancer, you are automatically at risk. From the Medical Intuitive perspective, this is true to a point because we take on our parents' behaviors and actions. This can cause the same effect in your blood as they have/ had. But this isn't the case for everyone.

So we live in fear of the unknown, wondering if we will end up just like them. We get a jittery, nervous feeling and immediately wonder if a heart attack is coming on. All we need to do is realize that if the behavior(s) of our parents is a part of ours and we haven't dealt with them, then we need to take a good look at them and decide how we are going to shift.

You know how we laugh when we hear someone say, "Oh no!! I'm becoming my mother!" Usually it's because we get that lovely "A-HA" moment when we hear ourselves talking just like she would or acting a particular way toward housecleaning, for example. The real truth of the matter is that we learned what we didn't like about our parents and vowed never to treat our children the way they treated us, right? So if this is the case, then when it comes to our attention, we will recognize it and shift it immediately as not to allow that part we didn't like to interfere in OUR lives today. This is important in how we see the word *hereditary* in our lives. Sometimes the behavior is harder on us than the disease! Also, be careful about judging yourself too closely. This can also have the effect of bringing it on because at that point, it becomes fear-based.

So hereditary bloodline comes from the energy of the reason a disease is there in the first place. Cause and effect are in action. This can always be changed, rectified, or even shifted in minutes once the "A-HA" moment becomes effective.

It's absolutely amazing today to have this understanding in transference. We need to remember that genes are just as mutable as water. There is nothing anywhere that claims that every single person will someday be doomed in life because of their hereditary background. If all things are

—

energy, then we could honestly say that we are in charge of this. My mentor of 12 years, who was a Cherokee Healer and seer of the body, used to say that there is no such thing as a miracle. It's just lack of knowledge. If you stop and think about that in today's world of Quantum Physics and Science, I believe we would find that true.

3.

DIAGNOSIS VS. CONDITION

"The simple truth is that generally happy people don't get sick."
~ Dr. Bernie Siegel M.D.

America is still a country that seems to be misdirected when it comes to health care. This is disconcerting when we can't even afford a co-pay, let alone a doctor bill. Some of us are even having trouble with paying our mortgage!

In the past when it was thought that doctors knew best, it certainly didn't seem intentional that doctors diagnosed cases that may not be what the patient had at all. As a matter of fact, it's happening today that more and more physicians are finding that patients have more emotional problems that relate to the physical ailment. However, the solution is still at bay for the physician unless they can solve it with a pill or surgery.

In my 25 years of reading clients' energy fields, seeing eight people a day for 15 of those years, I have found nearly 500 misdiagnosed cases. They ranged anywhere from a muscle sprain to a serious heart condition. Some of the cases were diagnosed through a side-effect from another drug.

I do not like the term "diagnosis" mainly because this word represents that you are now labeled. If people think that it's better to have a diagnosis, that's fine. However, it might feel better if we were able to see what might be ailing us through knowing rather than guessing. Bernie Siegel, M.D.

---

has often stated that doctors do not really know what is the matter with you, and to live life well, you are best to remember who the true healer is. Of course, it's you. There are so many alternative therapies today that can offer help and suggestions for healing, and these therapies do not have to cost an arm and a leg. With so many people without health care insurance or even jobs, for that matter, the time has come to allow for more understanding through simpler and less expensive means.

Diagnoses are sometimes very difficult to call. One diagnosis can have several different symptoms. As a matter of fact, there are so many symptoms that mimic each other that it's hard to diagnose with just one label sometimes. For example, a stroke has symptoms similar to a heart attack. In today's world, there are so many unique cases that even doctors are confused as to what label they should hand to a patient. Personally, many clients concur that these are conditions occurring in the body, and that's what needs to be seen as the effect, not the cause.

I worked with a neurologist for a few years who said over and over that people with headaches and migraines were the hardest to work with. He said there were many different reasons why a patient gets headaches. As a physician, even he didn't know the best remedy to prescribe. When I suggested to him that the patient is confused about making a decision and possibly needs to hear that, he laughed. However, I didn't find it a laughing matter.

That is why when I did hands-on work with my clients, they learned that in a state of having to make a decision. If a migraine would be persistent, I informed them that this is when you know what decision to make, but you just aren't making it. It certainly isn't a fault; it's just knowledge that I read and deliver. Nine times out of ten, the client not only hears it, but then allows the healing to take place because the cause resonates as the truth. Then the headache doesn't seem to come back. THAT is energy working through bio-feedback of truth.

We are going through a period of time right now in our world where to be able to *start* to heal, we can apply simple measures. Going back to our values, such as being a good listener, remembering that we were once in the same boat as someone else, gives us more room to understand and be compassionate toward our neighbor, loved one, or even co-worker.

A few years ago, a client on her death bed came in because the doctors she worked with couldn't find that she even HAD a problem! They just knew she obviously couldn't eat and keep down any food or drink. They ran several tests, of course, and nothing turned up on a scan of any kind. They were then baffled and told the woman's husband (after two months of her being in the hospital) that it must be stress. No diagnosis could be reached. She had had a car accident, landed in between the seat, and soon afterwards, found she couldn't eat without throwing up.

Her husband came into my office frantic, carrying her in his arms and pleading for help. She had lost 55 pounds in two months, being fed only intravenously. We had not seen these people in our clinic before. The husband said he'd go anywhere that could help her because the hospital just discharged her and told him to take her home and make her comfortable. "There's nothing that can be done."

I don't take "no" for an answer very easily, so I had him lay her on the table. I took one look at her stomach from a distance and saw she had a small bulge at the base of her xyphoid process. To me it was obviously a hiatal situation, possibly a hernia. So I massaged her stomach area. I listened as she cried, saying God was punishing her and that she must have done something wrong. I assured her God wasn't punishing her and that it could just be a small blockage that hadn't been located yet. Sure enough, the hiatal was like a rock and was cutting off her oxygen as well as her circulation and blocking the duodenum so that she couldn't eat. I simply massaged it in a downward position and had her take deep breaths. Her tears then slowed and a sense of calm came over her face. I told her she might try to eat watermelon and drink hot beef broth and then come back in a few days.

Three days later, when I arrived at work, a woman was standing at the door. I didn't recognize her. She was wearing make-up, her hair was beautiful, and this woman threw her arms around me, thanking me for saving her life.

"Oh, wow!" I remember saying and asked her if she kept the watermelon down. Obviously, she did, and from then on, kept anything down she chose to eat! Within two weeks, she was gardening and enjoying riding motorbikes with her kids!

When we are diagnosed with *any* diagnosis, we have no idea what's really happening, except to believe what we've been told by someone who, according to American standards,

---

54

should know what's wrong with us! After all, how else would we begin to recognize what was happening in our *own* body?!

It would be nice if we could self-diagnose, but we would need to be really in touch with ourselves to do this. Wouldn't it be even nicer if we didn't have to diagnose at all and actually felt symptoms occurring as a wake-up call. We could begin taking homeopathic remedies or herbs to help lessen the symptom while, at the same time, taking responsibility as we see fit. Maybe we could even consider that energy is a part of everything and therefore understand some of the ways our body needs to let us know that we have to take a good look at ourselves.

The physical body is our vehicle. It is also our mirror. We know this, so then why do we *not* listen when it speaks to us? Something as simple as our eye watering could be that we haven't cried over something that is hurting us emotionally. Nine times out of ten, we didn't know something was there in the first place to cause that kind of physical reaction. When we have a stomach ache, for example, is it just that we must have caught a bug? Is it possible that we have been going through heavy changes and not dealing with a situation that calls it to our attention?

When the body is sneezing, we automatically think that we have an allergy. Allergies are usually because of poor digestion in the first place. Maybe the body is just clearing out from a toxin that it came in contact with. Also, when we have a condition like a cold, this is not because we caught one. It's because we either needed a break and we knew it, or we were facing a confusing dilemma and felt overwhelmed. Not all symptoms have to be devastating if we consider everything has a reason. Because we are sensitive beings and our bodies are our vehicle, would it make sense then that this physical part of us would want to alert us to our deeper emotions?

One thing I really learned working in the medical field for six years was that everyone saw the body as a mystery and that it had to be something outside of us causing aches, pains, and headaches. God forbid, your first thought might be the "C" word! A blood pressure is an interesting metaphor to life. If we really understood that, we would be able to detect that the systolic number (the top) is about the stresses that are affecting you from the outside world: Your job, your routine, your kids always needing your attention, the frustration of being in traffic, for example. The diastolic number is related to the stresses on the *inside* that are not taken care of or recognized. This may include your concern for a loved one, being afraid of getting a bad grade in college, not fitting in with friends, or numerous other reasons that cause a "lesser-than" reaction.

Is life really a crapshoot? We simply are not pawns to some matrix in the sky with no cause. In all things, there is always a *cause and effect*. An action brings a reaction. This is common sense and science. In the same way, nothing ever happens to any of us *without* a cause.

Some of these causes are based with fears, which, of course, lead to illness, scarcity, doubt, and all the things that stop us from our potential. What I've noticed most in people is their fear of not being good enough. This is huge! I would say it stands first in the world of "pain bodies." If someone has money issues and can never seem to get ahead in their eyes, they feel they did something wrong. If they get sick, they feel they did something to deserve it. If someone sees that a person is whispering quietly to another, they automatically think they are talking about them. When a loved one dies, they feel, "Did I say all the right things?" It's the "Shoulda, Woulda, Coulda Syndrome." The list goes on and on around this issue. Truly, it becomes a self-created judgment, and it puts us in an awkward position within ourselves. If you think of how our cells mimic our thoughts and behaviors, then what do you think will or might possibly occur in the body when these questions are asked and not dealt with?

~ The Culprit: Insecurity ~

Through every person, there has been some form of insecurity that stands in our way of clarity. These are fears that become blockages on some level, preventing us from becoming free in ourselves. The opposite of this is confidence. Inner peace is what we are all seeking, and to get there, we must recognize what it is that continues these behaviors within us.

Even though insecurity is an expression of the lack of self-esteem, insecurity can be a TOOL when we recognize it, and it can lead us to the peace of confidence inside. It can be a stepping stone. It brings up sensitivity, which then can transform into compassion as we see ourselves learning through it. Being aware of our perceptions and recognizing them as such, we can change them in an instant.

We simply cannot escape the law of attraction, however, or the law of cause and effect. So I've listed a few of these behaviors to help us identify them in ourselves.

Here are a few insecure behaviors to ponder:

Denial, anger, lying, defensive behavior, manipulation, giddiness, control, unrealistic ideas, the all-knowing behavior, quietness, submissiveness, dependency, co-dependency, escapism, over emotionality (drama queen or king), over confidence, constant fatigue, complaining, loudness, irritability, overly talkative behavior, ego, anxiety, being opinionated, and being overly religious.

I'm sure you can come up with a few of your own. It's fun to teach a class on Body Intuition and then have students come up with what they see as insecurities. These are what they see in others that they wouldn't have thought about if it hadn't been presented to them. These are just some of possibly hundreds of corresponding behaviors resulting from a reaction to insecurity.

People who have come into their own understanding of power within themselves have noticed *when* they are watching the mirror in themselves through others. The psychologists say that we could be more observant of our Selves if we "see that what we don't like in others is what we don't like in ourselves."

Some would argue that point and say, "Absolutely not! I would never do something like that to someone!" Of course, pulling certain behaviors would seem ridiculous, yet we could benefit from being the Observer. My suggestion to everyone would be to become as aware as you can possibly be without judgment on ANY level. If we had only sacred confidence in our being, we would observe and become more compassionate, creative, factual, independent, happy, peaceful, understanding, non-judgmental, and positive. Mostly, we would be *healthy*.

The bottom line of truth in health for the soul is this: How you feel about yourself determines your own physical health. This goes beyond diet and exercise. Of course, diet and exercise are important to the body, but let's not lose sight of that which is sacred unto yourself: Your Soul.

~ Pointers for Healing ~

Here are ten pointers for healing that will help you on a daily basis:

1. Stay in the moment. This is where all power of life exists and creates the way of alignment with Universal Intelligence.
2. *Pay Attention.* You are the only one responsible for your actions, reactions, and non-actions.
3. *Be the Observer.* All of life is based on our perspectives.
4. Be careful in taking life too personally. It was meant to enjoy, not fight.
5. Be honest with yourself at all times.
6. *Listen* with more than your ears. See with more than your eyes. Insights and Truths can be gained through this allowance.

7. *Be aware* of your thoughts, your words, and your actions.
8. Quit blame altogether. There has never been a case recorded that anyone has ever healed because they blamed something or someone.
9. Remember that every moment you live, you are making a choice. How precious is that?
10. *Be gentle* to yourself. We all are learning how to expand our awareness.
11. Give yourself the space and time necessary to reflect. Beating yourself up won't heal the pain.

Below is a list I've put together that might help you in how to see blockages, on any level, that eventually restrict the flow in any part of the body. Blockages, such as the effects of our insecure actions, restrict the body's potential for healing. This can include blood, nerve, oxygen, and any forward motion toward a goal. These obviously cause dysfunction and discomfort as well. Here are some common themes I've read through performing energy work in others when it comes to conditions in the physical body:

Allergies: Blockages in the stomach and intestines. What are we not digesting?

Alzheimer's: Preferring the old ways over the new. Why can't things just stay the same?

Acne: Disgusted with your own self-image. Not sure of what face to show others.

Aching: Craving love so bad, it hurts! (Depending on where the ache is, the language speaks for itself.)

Adrenals: Overused and underpaid. Adrenals are the *fight or flight* glands that keep us going in stressful times. How much are we putting out and how much are we allowing?

Addictions: Lack of self-esteem and not accepting deeper meaning in life. Deliberate ignorance and emotional running.

Anxiety: Fear generated by past experiences not yet released.

Arthritis: Joints are related to this. Joints determine flexibility. How flexible are we willing to be? Not letting go.

Asthma: Fear from past lives, somewhat acknowledged in this life. Feeling alone, not safe.

Bladder: (cystitis) Being pissed off. "But this is all I know!"

Blood Pressure: What pressures stand in our way to freedom?

Bones: Past lives and memories stored there. Marrow is the meat of our past.

Bowels: The "outcome" of the day. Pressures either building or releasing.

Breasts: Lack (or not) of love and nurturing for the self. Left side: Am I allowing love into my life? Right side: Am I willing to give love? Am I possibly giving too much??

Bronchitis: Feeling that you can't change a situation happening that is close to your heart. Inner congestion.

Cancer: This brings up inner upset. Deep hurts unresolved. Anger toward self.

Candida: "Can anybody hear me?" Lack of trust. Deep frustrations not recognized.

Carpal Tunnel: "Why can't I make this life work?" It's a form of outward frustration relating to the nerves held deep under the armpit. This is also where we keep our deepest secrets so others can't see them.

Cerebral Palsy: A complex yet most loving way a person comes into this world. Loving toward family, and yet in a spiritual World. Not understood by many. When one of our senses leaves us, another gets stronger. In this case, the spirit over the body. CP is the most loving and spiritual condition. Anger and frustration come from "Why don't they understand me?"

Cold Hands and Feet: Not trusting yourself. Believing you may never "live up to...."

Colds: We simply don't catch colds. Colds are mental confusion. Not sure if you should choose one way or another.

Coughs: Not sure how to express your deepest concerns or fears.

Cramps: Not relaxing with the flow of your life. Feeling that there has got to be more.

Depression: Making yourself stay in a situation or feeling that you hate. Depriving yourself of happiness because you feel committed.

Dizziness: Scattered thinking. Confusion of the next intent. Sensitive instability.

Edema: Tears not released. Better to cry. Swollen emotions.

Fat: Oversensitivity. Sadness. A need for a way of protection. Where is all this weight coming from? (Can also be holding onto others' or your own emotions in the body.)

Fatigue: Boredom, resistance, and denying what it takes to move forward. "What's next?"

Fevers: Anger. Burning up inside. Emotions not released.

Fibroids: Questioning if you are loved. Nursing pains from the past.

Flu: Time out. This is your body's way of making yourself slow down.

Gum problems: Not making a decision for yourself and not sticking to it if you did. Be clear, and go for it!

Hands: Represent holding on or letting go.

Hay Fever: Not feeling that you deserve to be happy. A form of self-persecution.

Insomnia: Fear, guilt, and a feeling that "I just can't control life…"

Itching: Nerves encountering a situation left unresolved.

Jaws: Coping with life. "How do I do it?"

Kidneys: Disappointment. No real support. Feeling Unloved. Pissed off.

Lymph problems: Hiding your innermost feelings. Over sensitivity to an emotional cause and not dealing with it.

Muscles: Representing our ability to move in life. How flexible are we?

Nail biting: Not liking yourself and wondering if you really have anything to offer. Questioning your worth.

Nerves: Communication with yourself…or Not!

Parkinson's: Not learning how to give love to the self. Non-fulfillment. Overboard for others. Obligation.

Pneumonia: I'm so tired. Trying just isn't necessary anymore.

Sacrum: What are you sitting on? Let's get to the bottom of the issue.

Seizures: "I've really had enough, and I'm going to show you."

Skeletal: Past lives unresolved. Deep core cellular memory not yet acknowledged.

Spasms: Holding onto old thoughts when old thoughts are ready to be released.

Sacrum: What are you sitting on? Let's get to the bottom of the issue.

Teeth: Not liking your situation. (Because they are bone, it could be past life pain coming up for release.)

Ulcers: Not feeling fulfilled. Leaving a hole and causing grief.

These are only a few conditions with associated causes. When you begin to realize how this makes sense that the body is our barometer, our communicator, our answer to the recognition necessary to identify what we *haven't* recognized about ourselves, we will begin to pay attention. Then we will understand more of the communication our beautiful bodies are trying to share with us.

Pain indicates a condition due to an unresolved situation. However, if we do not want to be in constant pain, we must be careful not to allow ourselves to instantly feel fear. The knowledge of pain isn't meant to bring in fear. It's meant to associate something we might be missing in our conscious awareness. If we practice this perception, we will find that knowledge of the human body then becomes our friend. Maybe this is what was meant with the saying, "Be your own best friend!" I accept that one!

~ Something's Wrong, You Say? ~

Many people are still under the influence of believing in a concept that pain indicates that something is wrong and we need to see someone to identify the problem. I have seen so many cases of a client coming in with muscle pain, joint pain, or a diagnosed condition leaving the client immobile or inflexible. There's nothing worse than desiring to be active and knowing that your body doesn't want to follow suit.

In years past, our acceptable trained thought around health was either thinking we were doing something wrong or something could be wrong. As time continues, that is the past. The current trend in energetic medicine is about you, the person in the driver's seat!

By changing our perception of how our bodies feel, we can actually "hear" a cause if we listen closely enough. This, however, takes quite a bit of discipline and non-attachment to the pain through the mental mind. We can use the other bodies we have to co-create healing within. It is similar to hypnosis; however, we are conscious of directing an initial confrontation to what is going on that is getting our attention.

For example, if your arm is achy and it stems from the shoulder, by putting all of your attention on the pain, you forgot to use the other parts of your make-up to help you identify why that shoulder hurts. You could apply it with an emotional cause or a mental cause. You can even say that the Spiritual Body is at work nudging you to pay attention to how much you are putting out without the proper balanced energy to continue giving. If we say, "The weight of the world is on our shoulders" and then feel we HAVE to keep pushing, we learn that eventually the shoulder will give out. The idea here is to recognize that there are reasons for the body to talk to you and become the bio-feedback that you need to understand for your own motives, your desires, and your intentions.

Nothing is random. If it were, then there possibly could be no gravity holding us in place, and we could all be floating around. The word "random" seems to be overused and undefined. Therefore, it becomes a cute excuse used for a real situation that is part of our living at the moment we choose on any level.

I've heard so many people tell me that they are clumsy, and that's why they fell. Truthfully, they are going through an insecure time and not feeling really good about themselves at that very moment that they fall. Therefore, not watching your

—

step kicks in, and a result happens. "To every action, there is a reaction," my mentor used to say! Using the saying "Random acts of kindness" is sweet. At the risk of sounding like Sheldon Cooper in the *Big Bang Theory* TV series, they aren't random at all! They are intentional in the very second you make the decision to smile at a stranger on the street.

Sometimes we will find ourselves walking into something or stubbing the same toe over and over. I found through the read of the body that this isn't random, either. It's actually a pressure point on your body needing to be released to help one of your organs to free up, keeping the rhythm and flow going. Or it could even clear up sinus congestion!

In today's times, with all the changes actually seeming to be speeding up, our physical bodies are also trying their best to keep up with our subconscious thoughts. However, the subconscious is more and more conscious as we expand our awareness into realizing that we really are in charge on a higher level. That's why the integration of your thoughts and actions are being recognized sooner. You might just prevent a fall or some reaction to a cause simply by finding that you are taking responsibility for your self-esteem and putting your foot forward.

~ Our Responsible Awareness ~

"We are not victims of our genes. We are masters of our genes."
- Dr. Bruce Lipton

Way before our fabulous friend, author, and Cellular Biologist, Bruce Lipton came into our lives, I had already seen hundreds of people that were experiencing beliefs of themselves that were not theirs. They had been handed set beliefs on a platter without ever realizing that they did not choose them! I am very grateful that the door is opening you to the awareness of the knowledge of Jesus who said, "The truth will set you free."

Our parents only knew what they knew, and the concept of blaming them is absurd as we realize it just isn't their fault for all of the mistakes that we see they made. The problem arises when we see ourselves becoming like them if we didn't feel supported in the first place! It makes sense, then, that once we witness this or that action, we will catch it and, therefore, break the cycle. You are then telling the subconscious that this is bigger than you thought consciously. You are now going to reconsider and be humble to the fact that you never want to act that way again.

If we can see this to be true, then we need to take it a step further. If you look deeper, you will see that we are learning about heredity through knowledge of quantum physics. We can change our perceptions if we have a desire to shift them. Usually however, you need to be ready for that. In today's world, we're there. We are fed up with old

---

conditioning that obviously does not work for us anymore. We strive to be independent and confident. How wonderful that is!

Now, the hard part of our conditioning is that we were born into a society that told us what to think about our health. Therefore, you go to a doctor, and they immediately are going to hand you a form to fill out. The questionnaire will ask you if your parents had heart failure, diabetes, high blood pressure, et al. After answering these questions, you find yourself wondering if you also will have that, which makes the visit to the doc a little scarier. (If you didn't have high blood pressure, you probably might now!)

So we were, and still are, being told that a major diagnosis will run in the bloodline, and you too can have this condition that can eventually kill you. At this point, my observation is: If the condition doesn't take you out, surely the medicine will! Either way, it's absolutely important to know that you are definitely not a victim to your family traits unless you have similar personalities that create the condition in the first place.

Old belief systems are disempowering to your health at this point. You are responsible to determine how healthy you will be. Will it just be your diet and exercise that you feel takes care of you? Could it possibly be your workouts? (God forbid you skip a day!) These are all fine and dandy for keeping strong, fit, and in shape. Yet I remember hearing the news of a doctor in my town that was extremely healthy. He ran every day at lunchtime, and had a big family. One day he went on his usual run and fell over with a massive coronary that killed him in an instant. Shock and rumors traveled throughout the clinic. No one really knew what caused that, yet I suspected the running was too much for the organs in his body. The hiatal muscle crept up higher and higher until his breathing became more shallow, putting too much pressure on the heart itself.

Several years ago, a wonderful book hit the shelves called *The Hiatal Hernia Syndrome*. (I happened to be reading this book when this doctor had fallen over with his coronary.) As a Medical Intuitive hands-on therapist, I saw cases of a high hiatal way too often. What caught my attention was that many doctors didn't. The book was published by Davis University in Northern California where years of study went into this. What was profound was that the study showed 99 different diagnoses in relation to the hiatal being too high. It could determine the reason for a pain in the shoulder, a tickle in the throat, all the way to a heart attack. It definitely is significant of heartburn or "acid reflux." There are amazing effects of a hiatal muscle that worked its way up into the cavity of the lung, causing a protrusion into the tissue, putting pressure on the lungs, heart, and diaphragm. That means circulation, oxygen, and the capacity to breathe are all now restricted.

What is also true is that most of us have a hiatal that is up there, and fortunately, have not had to endure the horrific results of its turning into a hernia. Yet the effects are still shallow breathing and poor circulation. That in turn prevents oxygen, which stops the clarity of thought and, mostly, true relaxation.

If we learn how to properly exhale and shove the little muscle down from right under the xyphoid process in between the rib cage, we would have more circulation, more oxygen, and clearer thinking, along with 99 less possibilities of being incorrectly diagnosed!

The body has many wonderful ways of healing itself. It is in constant homeostasis. We are the ones who throw it off, mostly through a lack of true awareness.

~ Left Is Receiver, Right Is Giver ~

Many of my clients have had surgery based on the pain that comes from the low back. The low back is essentially the common place where people are insecure to their own support. The tailbone is about survival. In a person's being, if they feel they are not supported, many times the hips will go out of alignment.

We all have this from time to time, but a chronic situation is inevitably going to produce a result, as every action has a reaction. In this case, the left hip up can cause pressure eventually in a woman not only in her intestines, but also in her ovary or her bladder. It's pressure on the front as well as the back. For a man, it can be that he carries his wallet in the left back pocket, causing the left hip to eventually go out after a period of time, which in turn can cause prostrate blockages, urinary dysfunction, and even diverticulitis.

After a while, like in any situation, something's got to give. A doctor doesn't see this. They immediately know that you are in pain and many times only know to recommend surgery. So many surgeries are incredibly avoidable! Yes, a chiropractor can get it back in; however, it can go out again and again. Good for the chiropractor, but not so good for you. Knowing what causes this is important.

The left hip that is too high is a reaction to the receiving hip saying, "I can't take anymore unsupported action in my life. I refuse to accept it." So it actually blocks the support area by moving up and defending itself. The same goes for the right hip. The right is the giving side. When the hip goes out on the right, it is usually significant of the energy of saying, "I refuse to give out support anymore to others. So there!"

A diagnosis can only tell us the possibilities of an outcome, but down deep it can be an incorrect judgment and can definitely cause more pain in the long run. The body will enlighten you as to why it needs to share its opinion because it is your barometer. Just like if your smoke detector smells smoke, it will set off an alarm to warn you that something is happening and smoke is detected. The body and the area of the body also are those alarms. It will set itself off for you to recognize that it needs your attention.

When your dog is hungry, she gives you a look and demands then the dinner that she requests. You wouldn't think about not having your dog fed, your car taken care of, or your appliances fixed. Then why do we deny the pain that is the sound off that wants our attention? It's time to see the reasons behind the actions of the body, to which, by all standards of quantum understanding, we are not victims. Today we often hear, "There are no accidents." I support this through all of the body work I have seen. Nothing is random.

—

~ Taking Your Stand ~

Many years ago, I had a friend who did healing work out of her home. One day she invited me to come to her house and have tea and a chat. Agreeably, I went with glee, knowing that when it came to chatting about health, nothing could please me more!

She told me a story of a dear friend of hers that recently had passed of cancer. It was an amazing and true situation that we all could learn from on every level.

She told it this way: "One afternoon a beautiful Native American woman, after finding that she did not feel well, went to the doctor for a checkup. Her doctor did a few tests and came back to inform her that she had cancer. He proceeded to tell her that she had six months to live. At this point, the woman slapped the doctor right across the face and said to him, "How dare you! Who do you think you are? That is between me and my God. You have no right to tell me or anyone else how long we have to live!" The woman lived three more years.

Then one morning she woke up early. She called six of her very close friends, asking them to come over to her house as soon as they could. When they had arrived, she informed all of them that she was ready to die. Her exact words were, "Today is a good day to die." She gave each of them a hug and blessings. She then laid herself down and crossed her arms comfortably. Quietly, with much dignity and grace, she slowly slipped away. My friend was one of the people that had been at her house that morning. I was honored to be told that story, especially since I was working at the hospital at the time.

Many people go to a doctor and do not ask questions. They feel like they are at the principal's office at school and aren't sure what they are going to be told. Therefore, they usually take what they hear as fact and leave. Sometimes on the way home, they wonder why they didn't ask more questions.

Patients who came in for appointments always had their vitals taken by me before the doctor entered the room. Many had high blood pressure. However, when I applied the technique of visualization, their blood pressure dropped before the doctor came in. With their eyes closed, I had them visualize a scene of being in a field of beauty. This could be flowers, grassland, mountainside streams nearby, or even watching fish swim. By the time the doctor arrived, their heart rate had slowed, and their minds were calmer. The white coat syndrome was curable in minutes!

It's time to put responsibility back into our health. If we feel comfortable seeing a doctor, at least have the questions you want answered up front. If the doctor cannot answer them, you will usually go for a second opinion. I had a client who had pain in his hand and was sent to three doctors. All of them had a different diagnosis! One even said he had the onset of diabetes! *What*? Wherever he got that answer was almost as bad as when a doctor tells you that it's all in your head.

So seeing a physician ought to be like a job interview. This time, however, you are interviewing the physician. This also reminds me of a realtor. If a house that you are looking to buy might have a leaky roof, you would seek out the truth or even look at a different house. This is how it must be if you are to see a doctor. Use your common sense and see if what he tells you feels right. After all, he needs a medical diagnosis code, and what he tells you may generally be all he can see from where he sits. Working in the field was wonderful for what I learned; however, one thing I learned was never to be a patient!

4.

LANGUAGE BEYOND WORDS

"Solitary trees, if they grow at all, grow strong."
- Sir Winston Churchill

Perhaps you have heard the expression, "As Above, So Below." It's been determined that memories make up our very being. If this is true, then it would make sense that we created our own physical body. The way of living a healthy, more vivacious life for ourselves seems to be how we interpret our lives through perceptions and beliefs. More and more, we are recognizing that old belief systems are not necessarily true to our own soul. We have become challenged as these times in our world are shifting and changing. As time moves on, we are actually becoming more expanded through our mental and emotional bodies.

So how can this work in the sense of healing old crippling diseases? How do we see and know what is actually occurring in the body when we get diagnosed by a doctor?

First of all, we have to be willing to learn about it. Most people are so accustomed to going to a doctor and being diagnosed and treated. However, many of us have realized that a doctor just may not know why a condition has happened in the first place. Some of them are even willing to admit that! (God bless them.) They treat what they see and are not necessarily going to tell you emotional causes, et al. They simply cannot, and that is not their job. I feel it is unfair to blame an M.D. when we have just as much responsibility, if not more, for our own health as they do to help us locate a problem or give us a diagnosis.

I have been an energy runner all of my life, working to help heal many people, including children. I will never forget the little one-year-old child that came into my office with her mother. Exhausted and drained by her daughter, the woman was desperate for help. She came in for an appointment to see if I could tell *why* her baby was so clingy, extremely fearful, and relentlessly angry about her doing anything around the house without her constantly by her side. She also specified that her baby was born with a giant cyst on her left buttocks that the doctors were saying needed to be removed through surgery.

Well, in order for me to really check out this situation, I had to have the "permission" of the child! I had to be able to touch the baby somehow without her getting upset. So I had Mom sit on the massage table with the child in her lap. The baby was fine with that, as long as she was touching Mommy! So as I observed this behavior further, I realized that this little blonde baby would appreciate it if I tried to give her a crystal out of my collection on the shelf. I asked her which one she wanted. She pointed to a colorful quartz. I gave it to her and watched her as she slightly smiled.

As she was observing it, I sneaked my left (receiver) hand on her back very gently. It was OK with her. Then, with her still sitting on Mom's lap, I went down a little further on top of the diaper to see if I could feel (intuitively) the energy of the cyst her mother had told me about. Suddenly, my gut began to contract, and the grief that purged from this area had me crying very hard, as silently as I could because I didn't want the child to get worried or upset. I endured this massive amount of grief as I wondered how in God's name this could be so strong in a one-year-old baby!

I made myself look through the grief into the cause, which was not easy. I began to see her in the womb at five months old, and there was another baby there. Then that one was gone. I looked up at the mother and asked her, "Was this child a twin?" Yes, she was. The twin had died in utero at five months. In the meantime, this baby continued growing and waiting for labor.

This little one-year-old girl would have been the first to be born. As I saw the image, the emotion also translated into what I was feeling and seeing. In utero, the infants were joined at the buttocks. As the live baby continued to grow, the loss of her sister was transferring to her. She remained clear that she would carry her sister with her by manifesting a physical remembrance in her own body. The cyst was the memory of her sister. If the doctors would have removed this cyst, the possibility of this baby living would be slim to none. (I find the correlation interesting that the vibrations of the words "cyst" and "sister" are very prevalent here.)

Separating a cyst of this magnitude would have been devastating for everyone. Once this energetic knowledge became clear to me, I was able to counteract it with recognition and accepting the emotion that went along with it. This alleviated the child's pain as I took it on.

I continued looking at the situation a little longer, and the baby was still infatuated with the crystal. Thank God! I saw that this little girl was very intelligent. The color that fit into her self-confidence was purple. So I told the mom that she needed to buy her a dress right away that was purple with a big yellow flower. If she could find one like that, it would help bring her daughter into her own world, and life would ease up for both of them.

One week later, she came back to be re-checked. The mother walked down the hallway to my treatment room. However, the little girl was lagging behind her, not clinging to her. As I laid eyes on the baby, I was shocked. She was wearing a purple dress with a big yellow flower on it. I asked the mom where she got it. She told me, and said, "Guess who picked it out?" Wow! The baby found it!

Not only did the little girl quietly come into the room on her own, she was holding a *Pat the Bunny* book and comfortably plopped herself down to look at it. We all were happy with big smiles, and Mom finally was able to rest.

Stories like this one have been very common in my 29 years of energy healing. Now by taking a step further, we can begin to energetically identify the language our body gives us through physical expression.

Here is a simple list of how the body speaks:

Arms: What are you carrying and who?

Armpits: Storage unit of what we don't want anyone to see. (Emotional)

Breasts: Nurturing the Self (or lack of).

Back: Relates to stress, mostly questioning life in relation to support. (Who supports us, or do they?) Lessons on supporting ourselves through love.

Bladder: Emotional resistance to life. Letting go can be so very hard to do.

Calves: Moving forward. Not dealing with past issues or patterns.

Colon: Going with or not going with the "flow" of life. Not accepting change.

Eyes: How do you see life? Is it correct to your True Self?

Feet: How we walk in this world. In which direction are we walking?

Heart: Not listening to our *true* self through our feelings.

Hips: General support. When they slip out, it generally relates to an imbalance in how you are relating to life. Feeling the lack of love and support.

Joints: Flexibility to or in your situations.

Kidneys: Holding onto resentment or anger. Feeling pissed off.

Knees:	Seeing life as unsupported. Inside knee is community, job, friends. Outside knee is personal.
Liver:	Old past hurts or current hurts not being released.
Neck:	Flexibility or unwillingness to be flexible. Willingness to see different sides of a situation.
Nerves:	Sensitivity towards a situation not acknowledged.
Ovaries:	Very sensitive past issues about creativity. Guilt stored.
Sinus:	Confusion. Letting go on a mental level.
Stomach:	Carries recognition of the digestion of real life.
Swollen Conditions:	Tears unshed.

Not all parts of the body are mentioned. I am giving you only a summary.

The body speaks for itself. Sometimes it's a little more complicated. It depends on what, when, and how these conditions were revealed in the "As above" to create the "So below." For example, if we carry a thought that because our mother died of breast cancer, we may feel the energy of that in our breast, eventually it may cause the fear that then creates the condition. Guilt for staying alive after our parent has died can also cause us to deteriorate.

The body only responds to us. That is what it knows how to do. None of us are victims to a mystery. There is no such thing. The physical body has a good reason for everything it encounters. It's up to us to notice how it recognizes and delivers.

~ The Connection ~

We need to BEGIN with the simple understanding that our body is our vehicle. Just like a car, it needs to be maintained, cleaned up, tuned up, and fixed up when repairs are needed. (And just because it has high miles, it can still keep running just fine as long as we take care of it.) Therefore, the body parts are meant for clarity and precision in doing their job.

Not only do the organs have a purpose, but so do the limbs, the trunk, feet and hands, et al. They all represent meaning for us to comprehend. Energetically, they all have a metaphoric logic, if you will, to identify their meaning for you. Even though some of these parts may seem self-explanatory, such as hands are about holding on or letting go and feet are for taking us where we are going, they also have connected reasons to the rest of the body.

The head is a good place to begin. Not only does it hold our senses, but it connects to the rest of the body through the

---

spine and nerves and directs blood flow and feeds our stomach. The brain tells us everything beyond our wildest dreams! However, the energetic part of us intends to teach us that we are also led by the spiritual side within, to hear and listen beyond our ears, see beyond our eyes, know when a situation "smells fishy". This is what draws us to intuition.

The human being, no matter what you've heard, is not stupid by any means. Logically, the physical body cannot be deemed as stupid or incompetent in any way, shape, or form. It knows exactly what it's doing, and at the risk of being redundant, only listens to our perceptions and beliefs and then feeds the cells and becomes the physical body. As above, so below. So why do we feel we cannot change a situation within our body?

As a teacher in energy healing, I remember telling clients even back in the 70's that we are riddled with insecurities, which then cause a ricochet effect in the physical body. I have seen over 200 of these nasty critters lurking in the systems of the most wonderful hearted people. I have counseled and treated the body through the energy read of the insecurity itself.

This then is what the body relates to and hears, easing into a calmer state. True recognition and confrontation on an energetic level sets you free. When you hear it from someone, whether it be an energy healer or your best friend, it becomes bio-feedback through sound and understanding. It takes that recognition to produce a positive result just as Alcoholics Anonymous saying that you first have to recognize you have a problem.

Life IS fair in the physical body because it is what we chose at higher levels to experience in order to learn this time around. The best part is that we can change it right here and now. It simply isn't bad or good. It is our interpretation of why we are judging ourselves that causes the insecurity in the first place. Here lies the problem. On some level, subconsciously to some degree, we have become our own worst enemy.

My good friend asked me one time what caused fibromyalgia. When I told her the answer of the energetic read, she responded with, "I think if I had that, I'd hit you!" Of course, my response was, "Are you sure you don't have it?" Then I smiled and let that one go.

Any dis-ease we have that has created a form of pain or stress in our body has to come from our world in which we perceive it. This is true even if we find that we wake up in the morning with a sore shoulder and hadn't worked out the day before. Pain just doesn't show one day and release the next by accident. The body can't help but memorize an experience.

For example, let's say you are in a car accident. Sudden trauma occurs to the neck. This would be called "whiplash." The body's reaction to this whiplash would be instant trauma or shock. On some level, the body stores the memory of this like a computer hard drive. Depending on who you are and your idea of this accident, this pain may take a long time to heal. The blood that comes to the tissues during this trauma can cause edema and definitely make you feel stiff and unable to turn your head very easily.

Perhaps two years pass, and you haven't received any treatment for it. Your neck is still tight. You are living with it in every way. Or you may have gotten treatment with an awesome chiropractor. Pain is minimal, and your neck isn't so stiff anymore. Then you go to work one day, and you are told that you have a new boss. This boss and you clash. Your feeling is:

1. Shock that you weren't told this was going to happen.
2. Knowing that you knew you weren't going to get along very well.
3. Worrying if you are going to keep your job.

Suddenly you are faced with a situation to which the body resonates ....TRAUMA. Lo and behold, the neck starts to hurt. Then you have a lack of range of motion, and God forbid you have to take time off time to see a doctor!

This is a type of etheric biofeedback that is happening beyond your control. In a case like this, it's important to consider that you CAN shift this, and you must if you want to go on living without the idea that all sudden circumstances lead to pain from an old accident. It always amazes me how many people come up with some reason on their own to identify why they are in pain (what must have happened that the logical mind wants to believe so as to avoid the inevitable, the truth).

Of course, in spiritual understandings, even the car accident taught you something. It's hard to live life thinking we create our own reality and then have something like a car accident. Whose fault was that? If we could just remember that blame doesn't serve anyone and that whatever we attract, even as kids, is a part of the life we chose. We love to hear positive speakers, but do we really listen to them? Do we live what we heard, or do we say, "Yeah, they were good, but I'll never remember it all." Do we even refer after one month to our notes that we took?

What did we get from the phrase "The Law of Attraction?" Is there more to this phrase in life, or were we just hoping we'd get rich from it?

There truly are NO accidents. In every experience, we learn. If we didn't learn that we were taught to become better for obvious reasons, then why be living? Lessons are life, and life is lessons. In every moment, we own our choice. We can change it any time we want. Hence, we have the term PERCEPTION.

~ Becoming the Observer ~

When I was seven, I was sitting in our living room doing what a kid does. I was observing what it was like to close one eye and open the other and then quickly switch it by opening the other and closing the other. At this point, I was watching a change in how I saw what was in front of me. My mom watched me doing this and said, "Now what are you doing?"

I told her, "I'm watching different worlds out of each eye." Isn't it funny how we term our perceptions on how we view what we see?

If you've heard the term *Observer*, more than likely you've studied metaphysics for a long time. As time goes on in your life, you may want to be someone else. Many kids experience that feeling when they're young, wanting what others have because they don't like something about their own lives.

Believe it or not, this is usually how the ability to become the Observer occurs at a very young age. It takes something meaningful to pull a child out of their surroundings on any level (emotionally or mentally) so they don't get locked into only *their* world. The same thing occurs when a child has an imaginary friend. They seem to be just fine pouring a cup of tea for the party that isn't visible. We aren't. Many parents would like to discount that friend immediately and prefer to bring the child back to "reality."

I'm sure there are counselors who would disagree with me. I had an imaginary friend, but he wasn't imaginary to me at all. I spoke with him, laughed with him, and even thought he would send me messages at night when I was sleeping. I won a spelling contest in first grade and knew it was he who whispered the letters to me. When I wrote poetry for my mother at a very young age, it was he who helped bring in the words to finish the masterpiece. I felt like the quiet Observer as I accomplished these valuable connections because I simply paid attention.

I like to speak of being an observer in life, no matter what age. When my siblings got in trouble, I saw their actions and why they got a spanking. I knew NOT to do what they did, and this is a form of being an observer. I'm sure many of you can identify with me on that. When we know as adults the times to keep our mouths closed because our coworkers won't like the remarks we want so badly to make, we are the Observer in that situation.

You care about others and feel their concerns. Your baby cries, and you sense he's hungry. Your mother calls, yelling at you, and somehow you realize it's not *you* she's yelling at. It's the fact that she broke her favorite vase trying to arrange it for a dinner party that night. These are examples of being the Observer in life to those nearest and dearest to you. If we take everything too personally, it becomes selfishness on our part, and we negate a compassion that sits waiting for us to observe and then act upon.

When we reach a point in life, for example a midlife crisis, and we are aware that we might be feeling sorry for ourselves, we listen internally and suddenly realize "How will I choose to react to this emotion?" *That's* being the Observer. Being the Observer is basically a keen sense of awareness that you catch through yourself and through others. It's where you see life from a small distance, not to ignore it or even to deny it. It's a way to interpret a fact at that moment, to just be the witness. You are witnessing life as an Observer.

One of the reasons being an Observer works wonderfully is that you can see the big picture. The mind takes you away from the ego perspective and shows you an alternative to emotion. It gives you a fact instead of an attached emotion.

~ Attachment vs. Detachment ~

When you hear the word "attachment," what is the first thing you think? You might consider it to be a comforting thought. Some wonder if it's good or bad. Others will tell you, "That's my problem. I attach to everything!" We can even attach to attachment!

The truth I found in reading energy is this: It is neither good nor bad. These concepts do not exist in the higher realms of consciousness. We made decisions a long time ago to judge what we consider good or bad, but it really narrows down to perceptions and opinions of our actions and reactions. Perception is the true reality of our world. Attachment then is when we have made the decision to connect in a form where the ego lives.

A client many years ago asked me to read the energy of her sister. I had to explain to her that by Universal Law, it was not respectful or even allowed for me to read someone else's stuff without their consent. However, what I could do for her, the client, was to help her heal herself. That in turn would free her from the worry and fear that she had around her sister and her issues. I explained that we could help ease her concern that her sister might die.

She understood but then said to me, "So I'm not helping my sister by worrying about her, am I?" The sad truth was no, she wasn't helping anything. She realized after recognizing her fears that it was only transferring into the weakness of her sister.

This was a very important moment of truth for her. About a week later, I received a phone call from her. She called to tell me that her sister was now getting stronger, and even their conversations were better! There was laughter instead of dread.

We confuse attachment with loving. Attaching is a principle we use to help us feel like we have something close to our hearts. In reality, the closeness we feel can never really expand into a life generated by love if we deem it necessary to hold on through attachment. It eventually becomes conditional, and then we may lose instead of gain.

In the same way, due to our learning as children, we became attached to what we thought we *should* do...for our parents, our peers, or even God. In the meantime, we forgot to see through the eyes of the moment and experience our feelings from a clearer perspective rather than thinking we had to have an attached outcome. This is where we are today. The children of our time are much more aware that they live completely and honestly in the moment. They state how they feel, what they see, and where they perceive truth to be. Nothing can stop these kids from this enormous joy within themselves unless they feel stifled by an attachment of duty.

In order for us to be free thinkers and feelers, we must realize that independence is crucial yet know that oneness is a natural state of being. We can have a multitude of expansive communities of people who have a keen sense of this loving desire to work as a unit. However, for us to exist well and be well in this world, this must come from individual acceptance within each person. Then the community works as a team and not under the thumb of some system telling us how to do it.

If we continue to live by the standards of others' decisions for us, we are doomed to misunderstand the true concepts of living. In most cultures we do not have arranged marriages anymore for the simple reason that it wasn't our choice but rather one was chosen for us. I can hardly watch the movie "Fiddler on the Roof" anymore for that reason alone. However, that doesn't take away the love I have and for that sweet father played by Topol. You've just got to love his passion for his daughter's happiness!

Inside our bodies, the energetic language from the cells tells me that it does not desire confusion. More than likely, that conflict alone can set off many dysfunctional patterns that lead to illness. Today so many people are experiencing this state of living through chaos, inside and out. As we begin to change our thinking, we become unsure about an outcome, therefore creating havoc in our body. We may not trust ourselves or are afraid of what outcome may occur to a changing situation. Our immune system becomes affected by this because it is related to the nervous system. These systems in our body then become hyper-alert. Vulnerability sets in, causing anything from a common cold to an auto-immune disease.

If we understand that we can no longer hold onto the attachments of the past and have the courage to see this, then we will understand that the body will be releasing *through* chaos, as our world is also doing. Therefore, it is not a bad thing that this is occurring. It is a blessing so that truth can find its way in through these cracks of acceptance, and then we have light to lead us in the next step of our evolutionary process. This is what we call ENLIGHTENMENT and is ultimately where this world is heading.

We are not necessarily detaching. We are becoming more aligned to the oneness aspect of our true Selves. Our health is related to this configuration as oneness continues to become clearer within ourselves. It would certainly help if we could trust this process and do our best at staying in the moment, rather than fretting about the "what if's" that have not occurred.

5.

YOU AND YOUR BODY:
A COSMIC MARRIAGE

"If so much energy is in one beam of light, think of how much power one human has in one thought. All beings have the capacity to heal themselves." ~ from The Movie K-Pax

~ "As Above, So Below" ~

If you've never heard the term "As Above, So Below," it's a term I like to use to identify how energy works with the human body. Most people have heard by now, thanks to movies like *What the Bleep Do We Know?* that like attracts like, and your thoughts are things. Many authors today are using this quantum expression to get the word out on The Law of Attraction.

In the energetic readings I've done on the human body for over 25 years, I learned that "As Above, So Below" holds true to all experiences and thoughts in the past, the present, and even the future! "As Above" includes your mental body, your emotional body, and your spiritual subconscious. The "So Below" portion is our physical body. Your body is its own entity, mimicking your every thought, every experience, and every situation in a decision you've made or a feeling you've had.

The kicker is that our body knows us better than anyone ever could. It heard you. It hears your innermost secrets and your little white lies. It hears the excitement of a new relationship and the grieving of a death, even one that occurred 40 years prior. There's nothing the body doesn't know about you. It even taps into your subconscious mind and pays attention!

The term "As Above, So Below" is important to consider when talking about the marriage of you and your body. Many authors and teachers have shared their knowledge about the spiritual body; the mental body; and the emotional, causal, and etheric bodies. We have learned about how our thoughts are things and that we create our own reality. Rarely, however, have I heard people talk about how the cellular memory process works in the physical form when it comes to bodywork and the releasing of this.

In the experiences of my work, I have definitely come to the conclusion that _all pain is energy_. All parts of the body have something to say. It's like they all have their reason for being where they are and why they act and react to aches, pains, even becoming much more. Therefore, conditions (or as some people call "diagnoses") happen for reasons that are not seen or detected by an MRI.

As in the Universe, energy in our bodies doesn't know the difference between right or wrong. It just knows how to respond to an "intent." Our intent is our desire. The heart picks up this feeling and immediately transports it to the nearest port that has similar cell patterns with which it can identify. That port can be under the armpit (where people store their deepest emotions that they don't want others to know about) or perhaps in the thigh. (That storage place would indicate the support, or lack of, in you regarding moving forward.)

It can be anywhere, on any pressure point, or even down the spine. One woman I have seen was an actress, and her life was depicted through the apex of each vertebrae! Honestly, from the top of the spine (the atlo-axis) to the tailbone, she told her own story. I read from the time she was a 17-year-old looking for work, then a boyfriend/marriage, then her career, a divorce, the job, and finally, depression that had set in the tailbone! Whew, all this just in her spine! That didn't include the rest of the muscle memory.

This lovely lady decided to hang on to all of her feelings and literally to bury them in bone. People might do this because they don't want to forget their experiences and have decided to hold on to them. Even though we might think that's a hard way to live, for her it was the way she chose to learn spiritually. (Bone always represents past lives or past living.)

People store their emotions, mental ideas and wishes, and even their spiritual concepts directly in certain areas of their physical form. These areas can be in any muscle, leg, arm, et al, depending on a location where a trauma has hit or a place in the body that recognizes intensity.

If a runner who has run for many years develops more leg cramps, would this be due to the idea that the person is not getting the fluids necessary? Maybe it's a chemical shift in the body? Maybe it's that he is just lacking potassium? Could it possibly be that, in fact, the person has decided to "stop running" from life and decided to get involved?

Leg pain is usually about moving forward. Left side is receiving... on everyone. Right side is giving. If the runner begins to get heavy leg cramps on the right leg, the read might be that she/he is giving out too much from themselves and not paying enough attention to the need inside. Moving forward, then, has been ignored and has given the body the idea that "Enough is enough!" The person is then ready to stop running so much and get on with life from a different perspective.

~ Listening To the Body ~

The body loves when we hear it speaking.

I remember when I was five years old, my mother had lain down on the couch and had turned on the television to relax after 10 hours of working. I sat down next to her and, even then, asked her if I could rub her feet.

The look on her face was precious! "Of course!" she exclaimed. Then came the best foot rub ever, so I thought!

She did the cutest thing as I started rubbing her foot. She began to wiggle the one that wasn't receiving the rub at that time and acted like that foot could talk. Her expression was priceless when she began talking with that wiggle in her foot, saying, "What about me? Don't forget me!" So I put the foot down that I was working on and rubbed the one that was complaining. Within two minutes, she began doing the same thing with the other foot, then the other one.

Even though I was feeling like her feet were selfish and wanted me all to themselves, I learned at that time the body actually DOES talk, even though my mom spoke for hers! Little did I know back then, at five years old, that I would be doing this for a living one day and that I had learned from my mother about body talk. Your body definitely will tell you when it wants attention!

We have been told by science that we shed our cells on a regular basis, and every 11 weeks we have a new liver. After six weeks, we get new kidneys. After a few months, we are apt to have built naturally a whole new body! If this is the case, then why do we have chronic pain and continue to hurt, even at the risk of getting worse?

Every cell in your body has memory. Author and Cell Biologist Bruce Lipton has told us that we have five trillion cells in our body acting as a community. Either they get along and work things out or they have "environmental debt." When the latter occurs, they cannot replenish themselves fast enough to heal due to the beliefs and the power of our thoughts of being a victim.

Basically our bodies are storage units and have a lot of room for more. *Just because we shed the cells doesn't mean we shed the emotion inside the cells.* We carry this information like we're computers. We keep it in the archives, and then we can pull on it at any time we recognize that we are in a position to use it. For example, let's say when you were very little and baking with your mother for the first time, your father jokingly made a comment that you made dry brownies. At first you had been excited to see that your dad was going to get a brownie. To a kid, this is a big deal, right? Then he made a comment, even though it was done jokingly, and you were crushed. You didn't respond, but inside you felt you had failed horribly as a baker.

So when you are an adult, you are making dinner for a mate, someone for whom you want to do something nice. Do you think that old memory of your father's comment has left the body? I doubt it. Somewhere in there, you will be ready if your partner doesn't like what you've done for them. Chances are you might even feel defensive before anything can even be said. Expectations can arise that no matter how good you think you've made it, it won't turn out well. You also might think that you're a lousy cook and shouldn't even attempt to *try* to cook. But somewhere you will carry this memory until you release it and confront it. This, in a sense, is biofeedback to the cells.

Emotions are number one with this body of ours. Believe me, our body carries hurts, disappointments, trauma, and a lack of self-esteem or insecurities more than any other emotions. This is because the memory was harsh. The feelings of being accepted or not are huge within us. Other emotions are tied in as well but not as strongly as the harder ones.

Reading certain people's muscle memory is like watching the evening news! Each person is so unique, and what we choose to carry, to remember, is what's important for our health later on. The emotional body can create our physical template. Illness can certainly be attributed to our emotions even before the mental body has a chance to interrupt.

The immune system is the most sensitive for holding deep emotions and not recognizing them. Lymphatic action can result in confused states because we are doing what we "thought" we were supposed to be doing in life, perhaps trying too much to please others. Maybe on some other level that we weren't catching, we were angry. In a very sensitive system, a situation like this can result in lymphoma. Fevers are unexpressed hatred or deep anger. Feelings that we need to live up to someone else's expectations, or even our own sometimes, can develop into a serious auto-immune condition.

So it is "how" a person interprets an experience that can cause a disruption in the flow of life. That disruption, in turn, can cause a condition in the body called "illness."

Years ago I had a client who had a condition called "scleroderma," a very interesting auto-immune dysfunction. My experience with this read was that no matter what this person had told me in regards to the medical diagnosis and explanation (for which they have found no cure), I saw that his body was closing in on itself. It was like seeing him being put between two walls that were both closing in. Eventually the tight skin was going to get tighter, the chest would get more constricted, and the heart would be squeezed. Yes, this is a fatal situation.

He had heard about energy treatments and decided to try one with me out of curiosity. (By the way, the statistics for a condition like this are more common to hit women over 40, _not_ men at the age of 28. So it was highly unusual to begin with.)

The young man had come in with a slight attitude that didn't seem to me to fit his kind behavior the day I made his appointment. He seemed so sweet yet there was this edge. He got on my table, and as I explained that energy work could change certain responses in the body, he acted rather surprised. After a few minutes, we began.

His girlfriend was in the room with us, and she was an absolute doll. She wanted to help so as his partner, I had her hold his feet while I continued. He shouted out, "What is she doing holding onto my feet when I'm paying you?" I continued anyway and then explained that partners who want to contribute can help in the process because they care. His response was rough, and so I realized I had to tell him if he kept up this attitude, he'd have to leave. This startled him enough to get him to relax.

I asked him, "Do you want to know the reason for your illness from what I'm reading in the energy?" Of course he did. I told him if he continued to be like his father, talk like him, etc, he would not heal. I explained to him that his body was taking on his father's energy so much that his own body was resisting it and causing an inner battle.

He responded strongly once more by saying, "How do you know anything about my father?"

I said, "You did come to an energy healer, did you not?" Then I asked him, "When was the last time you played an instrument?" (This would have been hard to do when his fingers wouldn't bend.)

He said it had been a long time, and he missed it.

After he recognized that he had taken on large doses of his dad's world, his body heard the news and released it. At one point, I had to use crystals as a laser over his stomach to help release the stronghold in the aura. At that point, he gave out a scream and then cried. His girlfriend did the same, and of course, I couldn't resist tears as well.

He came back once a week for six weeks. Then he went to the health food store to get cell salts (bio-constituents of the tissue used to replace the minerals, etc. that we have lost or used up). After six weeks, he went back to have the test done to find out where the dis-ease was on the charts or a scale. If you are at zero, you get the news that you are in remission. If you hit 50, you're dead. When he first came in, he was at 27. After six weeks, he was at two!

Wouldn't it have been nice if the physician would have asked him if he'd done something different? With no known cure, I think this would have been a very good question.

~ The Emotional Body ~

Our emotions are usually the #1 trigger in how we perceive ourselves. They are what carry the thoughts of ourselves, and they certainly can be harmful if we don't rise above them. However, to deny our real feelings at the time is withholding information to the heart itself, and that eventually will bite you back one way or another. That behavior resonates to a blockage and then can create one quickly. This alone is what causes a heart attack. After many years of this behavior, we can die from ignorance and denial. So many people have put a callus around their hearts so as *not* to be hurt.

If we didn't have our emotional body, we would not even know what love is. Some still don't. However, the emotional body is what we are mostly about. We simply cannot know who we are if we do not learn from our experiences and our lessons. Actually remembering this can really help when you experience any difficulties. It makes the pill go down more easily, and then you can be much gentler with yourself in the process.

In the 1990 edition of the book *Bringers of the Dawn*, Barbara Marciniak describes through channeling that emotions are the conductor and the connector to our Soul. We came back to Earth in order to understand the actions and reactions of people and then to rise above their insecurities until we act out of compassion. (My mentor used to say, "You don't spank a baby for pooping his pants!") This leads you to a greater perspective of life as you realize that judgment has no place whatsoever in life. The lack of judgment is what creates Oneness within us all. The emotional body makes the most important decisions for you in your life. It is directly related to the heart.

Remember when I said earlier that pain is energy? It truly is on many levels, mostly due to emotions and interpretations from our own perceptions and/or insecurity. As we learn to let go of the painful words or actions of another, realizing we had a part in it or it would not have happened to us in the first place, the pain eases. We no longer have to depend on an anti-inflammatory (tears unshed) drug or a pain reliever to go on. As Don Miguel gently states in his book *The Four Agreements*, do not take things personally. What a gift we have in realizing this is very important. It also takes courage.

~ The Mental Body ~

In the mental body of our consciousness, we consider the mind to be our decision maker. Do we not think that this is the job of the mental mind? Isn't that why we were given a brain: To think? Just like in the Wizard of Oz, the Scarecrow was so proud to know he had been given a brain from the Wizard. Now he could think and be smart, when really, through the whole movie, he was already making decisions out of necessity and survival. We do too, no matter what our IQ score tells us.

The mental mind conceives of facts and belief systems. If we buy into religion or any idea that refuses to shift within us, this could not only stifle the process of growth in a true Quantum Universe but also cause a brain tumor, aneurism, stroke, Parkinson's, dementia, or even attract a coma! I mentioned my client with Scleroderma. If he had stayed in the mindset of his father's thinking, this sensitive man could have died very shortly of a self-induced auto-immune dysfunction.

The mental mind is extremely powerful. It can help us live, or it can kill us. If we believe in a placebo, our body will connect with the belief because we have no doubt that whatever we are ingesting is curing us or making us better.

One time a general practice physician I worked with tried an experiment on a patient to see if it would work for him. The patient had come into the office several times with complaints of a migraine headache. He would wait in the waiting room for a very long time, and even though I felt sorry for him, the doc was watching this man. He was watching his behavior this time because he had been in many times for the same thing.

Prior to this particular visit, the patient was given medication that he insisted didn't work. The time before that he got a shot and said the headache came back and that he could still feel it. So the doctor gave him a shot again, but this time, it was only water. He told the patient that this was the strongest medication that he could give him for a migraine headache. The doc also told the patient that if this didn't work, they would have to do an MRI to see if he had a brain tumor. (Nice going, Doc!) I stood in the room and watched as the doctor put the needle in his arm with a syringe filled with water.

I had the patient step into the waiting room and stay there for 10 to 15 minutes for observation. I smiled as I watched him lighten up and take a magazine out of the rack. I brought him back to the room and asked the doctor to come in. The patient explained that this one seemed to be working, and he noticed five minutes after the doctor gave him the shot that the migraine became less and less. We did not see him again after that. Placebo had done the trick. Was he ready to heal, or was he telling himself he would be good so he didn't have to get an MRI? Either way, the mind was convinced, and it worked.

We can have an idea that we insist has to be the right one, and by all standards of our mind, it must be correct!

When the mind is sold on something, it has a very difficult time letting go of that conviction down the road. It sometimes takes an experience to occur in order for many people to be shaken to the core and to shift their ideas. However, as our world continues to be affected by the magnetic pole shift, so does our mind also change. This polar shift is helping us in the "letting go" process, and it also will help us to initiate an entirely new philosophy. The strong beliefs we've had are much more expanded into different concepts and ideas instead of rigid, limited thinking. More and more we are hearing people say, "I changed my mind "as they have a higher capacity to listen to other people, loved ones, and friends with a more open and compassionate mind. Better yet, their actions speak louder than their words.

The mental mind has many forms to it. On a positive note, it stimulates emotions by simply allowing them in. It can sense the creative nature of the soul, search out talents and adventures, and make decisions based on logic, not panic. It can adapt quickly as a humble employee of the heart. The choice is ours with the perceptions we make.

When the mental mind harmonizes with the emotional body, our intuition turns into knowledge and trust. We react to circumstances based on the feeling in order to make the decisions we must make. All of this can happen with the proper sense of agreement between the two. Today it would definitely behoove us to allow the mind and heart to become one since, in 2012, our 5th dimension is all about unconditional love and open-hearted awareness.

~ The Spiritual Body ~

Today more than ever before in history, our spiritual body must be understood for the betterment of the whole. This is, in retrospect, what makes us or breaks us. We cannot deny that we are one unit, living and breathing as we think and feel. So how does the Spiritual Body play a part in this oneness? Does it mean the religion we believe and follow? Could it mean our understanding of God?

Truthfully speaking, in my work as a reader, it is none of that. Our Spiritual Body is the one within that acts and reacts to life. It's the Observer, the Over-Soul that brings in the desires, the questions, the choices, et al. This is our subconscious. Those who realize that life never dies and that we have been here before in other lifetimes ultimately can understand that this life is a continuation of the prior ones, giving us another chance at making our life better.

The Spiritual Body's total intent is to get us to oneness since there is no separation in the larger picture, anyway. It is a journey to be well recognized. For it is in the recognition that we collide awareness with truth, developing a big bang prospect and eventually bringing in a freedom of joy, bliss, and gratitude. If we see it this way for a moment, we will realize that together we are more powerful, especially from the lessons learned.

In my early days, when I began working as an energy runner, I noticed that in working on babies, there was so much more than what we see in a small child. The Soul of a child is huge, and in her/his own way, fills a room with "bigness." If one cannot talk or seem aware, before any conditioning takes place, he is that much more capable of actually **living** the Spirit within.

Clients I've had with cerebral palsy, or even multiple sclerosis, have these spirits that determine their lives, as limited as we perceive them. They feel more of everything around them due to a lack of body function. When we lose one of our five senses, the others become stronger. This is what happens to clients I've seen with CP or MS. Their spirits are more apt to define their world through energy and see for others a better way of living per se.

On the deathbed of a loved one, we see them slipping away in front of our eyes, yet what we don't see are the days before they die, when the Soul's energy permeates the room even when they sleep. Their Spiritual Body is awakening to its own truth until their need to be here is no more.

As time continues in this dimension of awareness to which we are awakening, we are in our own way expanding as we gain depth in our wisdom, allowance, and humility. Humility is not a weak behavior as we might have thought several years ago. Instead it is a form of releasing the feeling that we know so much and opening ourselves to more possibilities. It is the opposite of ego. Therefore, our depth perception increases, and our reality changes.

Not only will the Spiritual Body guide us to more intuitive coaching, but also we are more capable of seeing the "magic of life." It is as if we have someone watching out for us. We must remember as humanity, this is the most volatile time in history for us to be able to correlate our ideas, our concepts, and our knowledge and help each other in making decisions based on the best for the whole. This is done through individual acceptance of one's emotional and mental mind to bring in the balance of the whole person and then the whole world. This is what true health is and where I see each of us going. When the mind and body are aligned with each other, we call this the state of *being*.

6.

ILLUSION TO ILLUMINATION

"Losing an illusion makes you wiser than finding a truth."
- Ludwig Borne

I love the fact that there have been so many wonderful books out recently, such as *Biology of Belief* by Bruce Lipton and *Fractal Time* by Gregg Braden, which talk about the illusions that we have created in order to feel safe. These "science to Spirit" kinds of guys have concepts backed by science as fact, which has many people listening today. Isn't it interesting that even 10 years ago, we wouldn't have been able to identify theory over truth? When the movie *Contact* came out, it rose high on the charts. Why? Because it showed that when faced with the sight of the Galaxy, unknown to many even at that time, Jodie Foster's character had been so enlightened by what she was observing that she commented, with monstrous eyes and a look of amazement, "I had no idea."

Living on this planet, on some level we know that life is spoken of as an illusion because we can change it with the way we see our own explanations. Let's take time, for example. We set our clocks to the correct time, run our lives by the time, and wonder when we are running OUT of time! If you see from the idea of Sacred Sight, you can identify that time is definitely an illusion. We set up these standards in order for a communication to occur so as to "keep track." If you can see it from a different perspective, you will notice that time doesn't really exist. We created it. It's a lot like money. The idea always remains outside of our true reality.

We have placed so much importance on these limited confinements based as reality that we constrict ourselves to them and judge ourselves because of them. What a circus when you stop and think about it! When you hear phrases like "We're on Indian time" or "Hawaiian time," you know you won't be "on time!" I have found for several years if you listen with your inner abilities, you will wake up when you want to, know when it's time to eat, and trust your inner clock. A friend of mine who decided last minute to ask me to go to a movie never had the desire to actually find out "when" it was playing and would always seem to call me at that "right" time! I was amazed every time with his ability to know when to tune in and not be concerned as to whether or not we would be late.

When my mentor would ask me to come to her house, I would say," Sure! I'll be there around 4:00 or so." She would politely say, "Don't tell me what time you will be here because if you aren't here at that time, I'll be worried. Just get here in the afternoon."

Illusion basically is creating something either out of what other people say or from what we buy into from the television, and not even knowing for sure if what we are hearing is correct within our consciousness. Illusion doesn't know depth of self and certainly holds us back from knowing the depth within others. We can make up or say anything we want, but that doesn't make it the best for our growth and understanding. Illusion doesn't know how to alert us to a sense of urgency inside of us. It keeps us superficial in a world of outside influences and in hopes that we are continuously "doing the right thing" or "making right choices." (Even that is an illusion!)

Many of the illnesses today are created out of this kind of thinking. I guess you could say that both words start with the word, "ill." Therefore, if you become more conscious of what you are buying from the media, conversations, group meetings, co-workers, et al, you can begin to be your own witness in observing a greater opportunity to see more clearly for yourself, not for the sake of pleasing anyone else. What freedom we have in knowing that we can trust our own intelligence and refer to our own destiny as "ours" to be grateful for! This way of looking at your life will help in confronting the old patterns that no longer serve you or anyone else around you.

Health is created from depth of Soul-centered thinking and living. Sacred Sight has us feel the moment in order to react appropriately for our inner Selves. When we come from this place, there is no guilt, no denial, no need for judgment. There is a sense of knowing that leads to *illumination*.

Illumination is seeing clearly from an expansive perspective. I love the word "ILLUMINATION." You don't have to take a class in it. You just learn by experience that wisdom *is* illumination. The deeper you go, the more expansive you get. In the movie *What the Bleep Do We Know?* the question used many times is, "How far down the rabbit hole do you want to go?" That leads us into quantum physics and quantum awareness, but for now we'll stick with these simpler concepts.

I have had clients knowing that they "felt better" in their spirits when we were together, even though they knew they were going to cross over! What a beautiful thing to be with that courageous Soul at that moment! As the body was dying, the spirit soared, and the room filled with expansiveness. It was obvious to me that their energy filled the whole room.

One human body could not contain this due to our earthly existence and having to meet requirements and deadlines. Well, at the end, it IS a deadline, and the buck stops there. What a privilege it has been to experience that knowledge!

To the same effect, when babies come into the world, we see them as fragile. We see a helpless little body, and when we see the baby open his/her eyes, our hearts jump for joy! We are still, however, not aware that the baby is more alive than we can imagine. This child has a knowing larger than we can conceive and remembers more clearly, senses more strongly, and sees differently than we do. We have been conditioned. Babies have not. So even our understanding of what our eyes have shown us about these little innocent beings is an illusion.

~ Ways to Awaken ~

When standing in stillness, we wouldn't necessarily stop and consider the concept at hand called," standing in the moment of Truth." However, it's the desert that offers as many nutrients as the ocean, and stillness might be looked at like the desert. When we learn to turn within, we open and allow ourselves to become the change. Ironically, no thought has to be involved. JUST BE! This is where answers lie. This actually goes beyond ANY thought that you could possibly think would help your mind to ease or find solutions to a situation.

You will find that meditation is meant for this purpose. Dreaming is meditation on a higher level. When we wake up in the morning, we may feel different, even if we don't remember our dreams. The saying" She woke up on the wrong side of the bed" indicates an attitude observed that this person can hopefully realize. She then either will decide to shift her reality or not.

Our old patterns are being challenged now more than ever before. As we break through these old paradigms of thought processes and belief systems, we can trust (Oh no, it's the "T" word!) that we are opening ourselves to allow the shift to take place within us. We think we have learned so much. Learning doesn't come in one form. It comes from hundreds, moment by moment, and in these moments, the speed of light to illumination occurs. We just need to be silent and listen.

~ The Light We Are ~

When we flip on a light switch, we get results. When we get an "A-HA" moment, we *feel* results. Our intent of our desire around that keeps the light switched on.

All thought form is connected to an electrical current that runs deep within; it's the nervous system at work. This is what its true purpose in our physical body really is. The light we live is the power we are. By choosing the depth of illumination, knowing we have barely touched the surface, we can enhance our lives beyond measure.

Just think how much is out there that we haven't experienced!! For those of us who have been through the toughest of times, we feel we can say," Man, I can tell you a thing or two." However, what *didn't* you see in the reasons why you had to go through that tough time in the first place? There's always room for new understandings and growth. This is where we shine brighter. It's when we see more lessons for ourselves…minus the attitude. That is how we learn the lesson.

My daughter sent me a birthday card that had a Buddha on the front of it. Inside, it said "Have a great birthday and a new "Buddha-tude!"

That wonderful saying, "Once you've opened your eyes, you can't look back." If you should come to this situation again, you will recognize it and move beyond it. This process also provides you with the release of a pattern that has been there for a very long time. We all have known people, or even been someone, who continually repeated the same patterns, such as the same type of partner or the same lesson in job hunting. Maybe we have not been able to stand up for ourselves when we know down deep inside we do NOT like that job, but we take it because it pays well. In the true sense of the word, why would we spend a major portion of our lives doing something we know is in disagreement to our desires?

Temporary measures are lessons as well. Yet finding ourselves doing something we do not really enjoy creates a lack of energy that makes us age or begins depression. Even worse, it may cause a cancer because we stayed with something we truly hated down deep.

Illumination is clearly about waking up and changing the perspective from how we've seen things to being open enough to find how much more we haven't seen. In the movie, *The Matrix*, could Neo have known he was the "Chosen One?" Chances are, he couldn't have until he proved himself and moved out of fear. What does the term "chosen" mean, anyway? Doesn't it always come down to our decisions of how far we are going to lead ourselves without the blockages of insecurity? I wonder if Jesus or Buddha would have considered themselves "chosen."

Waking up is not just with thought even though we have a thousand thoughts a day. It's about stepping out of a blockage of time and limitation that we have created and reconsidering a new direction. This can be with the comments you make, the choices you're making minute by minute or on a daily basis, or even your choice of a profession.

We are in a brand new period of time. The collapses and shifts all over the world are speaking directly to us as a mirror. It is truly time to "let go" and go with the flow of New Creations! To stay healthy we must remain in balance. In the movie *Avatar*, we saw that Nature's first priority was balance. In the physical body, we call it *homeostasis*.

The saying "All things in moderation" also relates to our emotional responses, our mental concepts, and our very ideas. We can achieve this balance inside ourselves, no matter who we are. We just need the virtue of listening. Listening requires patience. It requires silence. It IS the going within that brings about a sense of serenity and calm. Simple actions are loud. It helps in our healing by creating room for the cells to shift into a more expanded and accepting energy. This alone can change your frequency to allow a higher insight to occur. This is the ticket to how we create balance inside on a deep level. When we can listen and not be or feel threatened to "what" we are hearing, that's moving forward.

Standing up for oneself is truly happening with or without another person having to know it. Many times I've seen what others are like due to insecurity. (It's my job.) It's then that I get quieter and listen. It's like a patience sign in my mind goes off, and the sign flashes in neon lights. This person might appear strong when they are really scared. (This affects the circulatory system and is where the expression "It made my blood boil" came from.) They may act shy when down deep they have a lot to say (throat chakra effects and immune reactions). They may be feeding me information that I can read is just not true for them, yet this is where their comfort level is. Listening, patience, and factual perceptions have worked for years when Spirit has something to say!

~ The Age of Innocence ~

A child of one of my clients is five years old. She was watching TV one night when her daddy came into the room to put her to bed. When he told her it was bedtime, her quick response was, "Daddy, there is no time."

He said, "Then what are we doing here?"

Her response was, "You know this father-daughter thing? Can we just be friends?" Children are like Shamans in small bodies. In so many cases that I've seen, they are waiting for their turn to be heard.

At the ages of five and six years old, we are developing our sense of awareness to the big picture in which we are living. It's not that we lose our sense of Soul. It's just that we then have to define our system of how we are going to survive in the world into which we came. However, many children today only have the moment. They do not necessarily think about going shopping for groceries, where their next meal will come from, or even when tomorrow will be here. Why would they? They have a sense of time that in the moment, they are making their reality happen. This is why the memories of a tot that age will be more significant in later years. They were there, truly present.

If the pain in the adult life is strong, so many times it's because as children, we felt who was there when the fever hit. Who helped us ride our bikes? If your memories were good and you had a loving family, you will remember your Christmas mornings or the smell of dinner that your mom cooked when she made your favorite meal. Memories determine your future. Whether positive or not, we usually allow them on a subconscious level because that's all we know.

Many people are talking about living in the moment today. Actually, it's Quantum Physics that taught us that there is NO time, and there is only that which we create. If this is true, then the good news is that we can change the memories that we created just by not attaching to them as reality, especially if we hold onto them and determine the rest of our lives by them. This is why there is hypnosis. To really dive into memories can heal us, and it can also hurt us. Those clients of mine who are aware of very hard or sad memories can determine their future through allowing the release of the importance of that memory to exist.

I had a client who had lost her mother at the age of three. It was she and her sister who lived with their dad. She always wondered what it would be like to have had her mother there. So we played a little trick on the mind. As I ran energy through her body, I suggested that she see her mom there during her years of important life events. Even though she could not bring back her mom physically, her mind saw her mother there and eased her into fulfilling a moment that changed the way she had felt all of these years. Loss and sadness in regard to this turned into saying, "It's like I feel her presence again," and that changed the way she interpreted life as a mother herself. It was in her perception. We can all see what we want to, and the feeling is what heals us. In her case, it was the satisfaction of feeling the release of that constant pain and wondering turning into comfort, nurturing, and love.

Can we change the past? Yes, inside of our hearts, we can. Our thoughts create the power (fuel) that feeds the cellular pattern. We are certainly capable of changing it at any time. Can that change the future? Certainly it can. Time and space are only significant to *us*; therefore, we can change it in seconds just by mere allowance of a new perception. This, on many levels, is why age itself is not necessarily the reason we die. When we are at an older age, and we have been healthy from all aspects in life, our organs can give out, of course. However, for the most part, we reach a stage in life where we can now actually advance and *move on* by what we call "death." Even in death, our perceptions can lift us into higher realms of frequency on the other side. Again time over there doesn't exist. The more we are able to let go of this linear thinking, the freer we become.

When swimming with dolphins on the Big Island in Hawaii, I caught the eye of a mother with her baby right alongside of her, mimicking her every move. Her eye said to me, "We're connected," so I followed them. What I thought was only five minutes of swim time next to them turned out to be 45 minutes! Finally I realized that I had swum so fast, and when I dropped back to our earthly reality, no one was out in the ocean where I was! It is a fascinating experience when you realize that you were basically taken into a consciousness where there is no space or time. It was as if I were flying, and I lost all sense of direction and time. I didn't even care whatsoever.

There is not a thing that is set in stone, no matter what your belief systems are or for that matter, how you perceive anything. This is why being open and living every day as though it is totally new, is a "free-way" into being! People have asked me if a baby is waiting in the wings before a pregnancy occurs. I don't like to burst anyone's bubble, but with all the reads I've done, the answer is "No." It is not until a Soul decides to enter that the decision becomes reality.

We as humans do not see beyond our physical realities at times so when we try to understand the process of how life works, somehow it feels better to categorize it or say it is a certain way. We think we are at the mercy of a situation happening TO us. If we trust the power of the energy within us, we can shift it. Illumination includes spontaneous moments and allowance for something new and different to occur in any given situation. There is the joy and the adventure!

I will tell you about an experience that happened about 12 years ago when I was working. A woman who was five months pregnant came to see me. Her mom was a regular client of mine, and fortunately she sent her daughter in for a session. This daughter had not been pregnant before. When she came into the healing room, little did we BOTH know what was going to happen.

I asked her if she had ever had an energy session of any kind. She said, "No," but she had decided it sounded pretty neat with what her mother was experiencing in her sessions with me. This gal drove quite a distance for this session. As I started working on her stomach, I immediately read that there was no life in this baby. I asked the woman how long it had been since her last checkup. Her answer was, "Two weeks ago."

At this point, I looked up to the heavens and asked, "Why did you send her to me?" I then felt the need to put my hands on her belly, one hand on the baby's feet and the other on the head. My hands practically moved themselves into the position necessary for me to run the necessary energy. Even I wasn't sure what would happen here. The energy from my hands began not only to heat up but to permeate dramatically through this lovely lady who was seriously conking out fast! This was good. For whatever was to happen, the energy was acting to a degree like an anesthesia.

As I sat with my hands in this position, I felt a major surge go through *my* body! It felt like I was knocked off balance and my equilibrium took a few minutes to get back.

Within about two minutes, I felt a kick from this little baby directly under my right hand. I felt a huge sense of relief as the mother then said in a groggy voice, "Oh, there it is." Shocked and elated at the same time, I continued as though nothing big had just happened. I certainly wasn't going to blurt out, "Hey! Now your baby has a life!" This was a miracle, a moment in time that only I knew. Well, that Soul and I knew!

I finished the session, said goodbye to my client, and then went to the restroom to find myself strongly feeling a sense of sadness. I began crying pretty hard. After five minutes, I dried my eyes and started on the next person.

A week later, I went to have my own session with my wonderful Cherokee mentor. I asked her to tell me what had happened as Karen could read energy no matter what it was. She told me that one of my Guides had surged out of me and into the baby's body so it could live here now. No wonder I cried so hard! Losing a Guide that quickly left me feeling a bit weak and empty. I was told by Spirit that I would not be able to see this child in this life. I had the opportunity seven years later when my original client found me in my new location. She had informed me that the little boy was doing well and that the energy I had read during the session of this baby all happened. His labor was difficult, and yes, he was a piano player.

When I sneaked in the question as to whether or not I could see him, she said her daughter lived nearby. She would tell her I was at this new location. I felt hopeful. Yet, if he would have seen me, it would be obvious the boy would feel very drawn to wanting to come home with me. Maybe that would have disrupted their lives. Spirit was working in our favor when I realized I would not see him this lifetime. As sad as it made me at the time, the cycle of life had its own fabulous plan, and I was blessed to be a part of it.

So the age of innocence is about humility, spontaneity and adventure. This story I just shared is a humdinger yet it depicts how precious and special life really is. How these incidents happen to (and with) us becomes a type of miraculous event that we ourselves never could have imagined. This is the trust, the childlike allowance that we desire. These types of surprises in life are a form of answered prayer. If we have asked for more to happen in our life, this is the type of answer the Creator gives us. It's always through the movement and the enjoyment of life. Sometimes they are wake-up calls to attract and accept more. Therefore, the age of innocence can be said to be inside of us to allow, become, and trust in the love of the adventure.

7.

QUANTUM AND INDIGENOUS: FACTS AND KNOWLEDGE

"Humankind has not woven the web of life. We are but one thread within it. Whatever we do to the web, we do to ourselves. All things are bound together. All things connect." - Chief Seattle 1854

I am not a scholar in Quantum Physics with a degree in science or quantum mechanics. All that I have learned has been from "hands-on" experience and BEING that which these scholars talk about. With the understanding that we carry grids of memory in our very own blood, our bodies, and our remembrance of the past, we must truly know that there is nothing stopping the flow of this connected knowledge to *anyone.* We are simply re-remembering information that existed somewhere in our blood many lifetimes ago. Energy begets energy. Therefore, we are inherent with memory as we come back to this world to begin again the lessons of growth in order to achieve a higher frequency of living, a better life with wisdom. Transference, osmosis, conscious creation, and evolutionary patterns from the past are all part of us and our growth.

When I was in my early teens, I watched a program on TV that related to the queen of Mongolia. She was buried in a valley in the hills of Mongolia with 12 horse heads surrounding her grave. I do not remember who was digging up the grave; however, it didn't seem to matter. The point was that my soul almost jumped out of my own body because it was so auspicious to me. My skin developed goose bumps, and my memory recognition kicked in. I began to physically have a reaction, recognizing that queen to be me. I literally became aware of the knowledge of who I was at that time.

Since I am a reader of energy and have been my whole life, this sent me into a chill and shock to my current system. So instead of becoming afraid of it, I became one with it and read the memory of her bones as they dug up the grave and opened the coffin. I saw the jewelry that was familiar to me. I also was able to determine why they buried me there. It was sacred land, and I was well liked and respected as their queen.

Many years later, when I met my mentor, Cherokee seer Karen Land, I did not speak of this. Instead, I had asked her about my past lives. Our conversation was so real and so very resonant to my being. She told me that I had been a Mongolian queen who was buried with 12 horse heads around my grave.

One life always leads to another. I like to consider this life like a calendar. We turn the pages, but it's the same year. Each day can also be considered a lifetime now with how fast things seem to be moving! The Shamans know that there is no time and that one life leads to another to continue the process of undeniable desire to get to return to Spirit one day, whole and complete.

Quantum reality is based in true awareness of fact when science tells us that it's the space between the cells that carries the essence of life and actually dictates life into form, which is the cell. It becomes a virtual fact that these spaces hold the memory of all things happening in the body, and the cells become the conduits in order to perform what that information is. This is why we have the right and the means to change anything in ourselves any time we choose, just like having a genie in a bottle.

Not everyone needs to know their past lives. However, if there is a block in the current growth, chances are it might be a little harder than originally thought to advance. This is why we must be honest with ourselves through our emotions. This is the best way to advance. Again, where two or more are gathered and confrontation through growth occurs, we can step into a new awareness and see life as a huge chapter being written by you. It isn't so much the necessity to rediscover where you have walked. It is to be face-to-face with a lesson waiting to teach you the essence of the bliss you desire today, giving you permission to become enlightened through humility and expansiveness. This is the key to happiness.

A four-year-old child came in with a fever. He was incredibly smart and very cute. We spoke of this fever, and I told him I would be speaking to him like an adult. I explained his fever was about the anger he was carrying due to his brother not loving him the way he expected he should. He looked at me with those big beautiful brown eyes and said, "You are right on." I had him explain to me what he thought his brother should be doing differently.

Once he got the feelings out of his system, we talked about how his brother needed a little space, but he didn't love him any less. As I worked on his little body to get the cough to alleviate (Congestion is due to confusion about how to feel), he looked at me and said that he could only imagine how fun things would be very soon. I applauded this little sweetie and reminded him that as long as he didn't forget to see the reason *why* he got sick in the first place, he would get well and have fun.

I gave a talk on "Health Care for Today" recently when a lady from the audience came up to me and called me a "Quantum Shaman." I giggled and then decided that the title was appropriate, considering the understanding of cosmic correlation between our Spirit and our physical body.

~ The Prophet in You ~

Prophets of the past have been able to read the future. This is truly special and highly unique to those times when Nostradamus was alive. You can't have prophecy or any read without accepting the larger picture that there is so much more that we are now tapping into. These prophets knew this.

The truth is that *anyone can do this*. People believe you have to be born gifted in order to produce wowed effects. This simply is not true. Many people are coming into more of their own wisdom and hearing themselves saying things to other people that they didn't even know they knew. All it takes is pure desire and less negative talk about themselves and others. This alone changes the old patterns that have not been recognized by us and keeps us more open to possibilities with ourselves. It is as if we are emptying the bucket and cleaning it out in order to retain more. More and more people are also beginning to see that they recognize places that look familiar on some level even though they have not been there in this life. Many of our children born today are mentioning this to their parents without any hesitation.

The indigenous healers and Shamans have always known that there is no stopping the flow of God or energy that they accept as Oneness.

The only ones who stop any form of creation are us.

We have the free will to see things however we want to, limited or not. The choice will always be ours to allow or disallow. The more knowledge we accept as possibilities and truths, the more we let go and make it happen. The Shamans embody truth in themselves in order to produce truth in others. They don't have to say a word. They just are. Their presence alone fills a room with a feeling of awe and even hope.

If you've ever attended a powwow, then you know the purpose is for celebration and connection. What better form than dance to describe and express every cell appreciating life? This is respect at the highest level. Trance states have certainly been reached. I have seen some dancers that continually dance in high temperatures with all the regalia for hours and hours at a time. They are immersed in a trance state that allows them to keep going. Their intent is strictly love beyond their own ego. This transcendence overrides the fact that their bodies are so tired or so hot. At that point, they do not give that any relevance, and they just keep going. Their gift to their Creator is that of oneness in and throughout their blood.

When you walk into a place where there are elders, you naturally feel the respect throughout the area. We have had the 13 Grandmothers appearing for many to witness as they travel around the globe. What is their message? Peace and truth to all. They are providing a wake-up call to humanity, bringing their intentions through song and healing and prayer. The ancients are being acknowledged today for their sharp wisdom over thousands of years. If we didn't find this of any interest, then why would there be all of this commotion about the "end of times as we've known them" on December 21, 2012?

In the world known as "Indigenous," we automatically think of traditional tribes performing rituals to suit their beliefs and their way of connection. It is true, however, that the Shamans of these tribes become much, much more than *only* a part of his or her tribal connection. They become a light to the world through the oneness of their Spirit *to* the Earth and with the Divine. It is where Humanity is going.

All of us are being called on a deeper level to expand within ourselves, and it is definitely creating a sense of Unity, called Consciousness. As I say to many people today, we are now "Shamanizing Humanity." The calling within us is demanding us to break through the old paradigm from which we learned.

If we stop and consider that our learning has been based on limited concepts from others, then maybe we can trust ourselves in the midst of chaos by allowing the breakthrough to occur with grace. That means judgment must stop, and expansion must take place. We can all become like the Shaman by healing ourselves first. Then we can be more of a teacher, a supporter, and a healer for others. If we do this consciously, we have connected to the Spirit within us. This is why the Shaman understands truth. It comes from allowance, acceptance, understanding, and compassion. It's from there that the strength within gets tapped on the shoulder for more insight to occur. Trust is essential.

~ My Story as a Shaman ~

I have been attracted to, lived with, seen, worked with, respected, and loved Indigenous Medicine Shamans most of my life. Since I can remember, I have wanted to be an elder. I sat with my mother on the porch one day at the age of seven and said to her, "You must be real happy at your age."

She gave me a curious look and then replied, "What do you mean?"

I told her I wanted to be her age and get the benefits of discounts on groceries, et al.

She laughed and then said, "You are one weird child!" I just smiled.

I remember watching a movie on TV about Jesus on the cross when I was five years old. I couldn't take my eyes away from the TV. I sat practically right ON it when my mom asked me to scoot back. I told her," I know him."

Of course, she responded with a statement of how absurd that was.

My response back to her was, "Do you know how he stayed alive for three hours up there?"

She said, "No, smarty pants, how *did* Jesus stay alive for three hours up there?"

I replied, "He knew how to move his feet." I immediately knew that he could move his feet to keep the circulation moving. Even with a nail in them, that kept him alive for the time he had.

After those "A-HA" moments, I began to realize that I came back to Earth to do the work I chose. When in Sunday School one day, I looked down at my hands and couldn't believe how wrinkled they were at the age of 10. I noticed my teachers' hands and other ladies' beautiful hands, even my sisters'. Why were mine so wrinkled? I received information at that moment that they were very old hands. When the teacher said that Jesus touched people and healed them, for me, this was a confirmation. These hands had lot of work to do. So I accepted them and agreed they were OK. "Yes, they'll do just fine!"

At 19 years old, I heard of an organization called the Jesuit Volunteer Corp from my dad who did business cards for a priest in San Francisco. I was so happy to be accepted, even without the mandatory degree they requested with the application. I was chosen to be an Activity Director for four senior citizen centers in Juneau, Alaska. My experience with the Klinket Indian shut-ins was extremely gratifying. To sit down at the age of 20 with these beautiful people and listen to their stories was beyond what I ever could have read in a book. They shared their Native way of the heart, and they were so real. I didn't want to leave them. I'd come back with food, driving the "senior limousine" the next day and do it all over again. This went on for a year.

The day I got married, I had received a package at my door. When I looked to see who it was from, it was one of my favorite and wise Klinket elders who had taught me about what it was like to be blind. She died two months before her daughter had found the package that had been addressed to me. It was incredibly touching to know that I had made such a difference in her life. I felt that she didn't die at all! She bought me the towels I had commented on the last time I had seen her. She was gone, but not really.

Years later, I was introduced to my mentor, a Cherokee Seer and amazing healer, Karen Land. She had been recommended for me to see from a friend who had heard of her awesome ability to run energy in the body. Being curious, I made the appointment, and my life has never been the same. I was fortunate to have learned from her in every way for 12 years. Her wisdom touched hundreds of people, and the truth through her hands is where I learned much of the knowledge I've gained. When she touched you in your appointment with her, the energy in them was so high that your body would shake. Her hands wouldn't, but your body would. The feeling was so unusual and yet incredibly satisfying through the love, you truly felt at peace in a matter of minutes (regardless of what you were going through at the time).

I asked her once what the Bible meant when the Book of Revelations spoke of the "beast." Who or what was this beast? Her answer, simply stated, was, "Well, honey, the beast is the ego." That was enough for me. She was quick, sharp, and took me on as her student 24-7. The statement of the ego intrigued me. Coming from a Catholic background, this statement had me pondering immensely. As I continued to identify with it, more knowledge just kept pouring in. I began to feel as if I really understood what was causing humanity's suffering. It was insecurity and blockage of buying into hierarchy from all these years of control and manipulation. It made sense then to acknowledge that. From that moment on, working on individuals became easier. When we "get it" and an A-HA moment sets in, our lives expand and change. No longer do we have to buy into the idea of something "out there "running our lives. Just knowing that the ego was the beast made all the sense to help people turn this around. I always give thanks for that knowing from Karen.

When she passed in 2005, I had developed the symptoms of her last physical condition in *my* body, and I knew I needed a Shaman to be high enough in vibration to help rid me of this. I had a client at that time that was so grateful for the work he'd received that he and his wife sent me a first-class ticket to Hawaii. I had wanted to go to Hawaii for so long and never found the time or made the time to go. Through this wonderful client, it happened when I most needed it.

When I went to Hawaii to stay with them, I asked him if he knew of any Kupuna (a wise Hawaiian elder with the gift of healing hands) in the area. Fortunately he did, and meeting this Kupuna was the beginning of my knowledge with the Sacred Hawaiian healing and tradition. I studied under him for almost a year as an ala kai student to this sacred healing. Lomi Lomi wasn't just a form of massage; it was the way in which a true Hawaiian elder was able to interpret or see the body and work on many areas of dysfunction. I realized this must have been my life before because I automatically did this in my work from the start!

I found so many Massage Therapists on the mainland could not explain this meaning, no matter who I'd ask. They stumbled at their own responses. It wasn't until I found the beauty myself in what this meant that the answer was given. In Hawaiian healing, there is the knowledge of the plants and herbs such as the ti leaf. Each plant offers something, and it was the ancients that knew the benefits of them. It is the study of "Lapa au" (herbs).

These deep Shaman healers ("Kahuna" to some, even though that word does not have the same meaning as it did years ago) understood that greeting each other was most respectfully done with the "Ha" breath. This is a greeting given from Hawaiian to Hawaiian in the form of breath to each other. Two Hawaiians will put their foreheads together and make the exhale into a whisper of "Ha." They won't usually kiss at this type of greeting. It becomes the meaning of love, caring, respect, joy, and long life simply in one breath. When witnessed, it's awesome! This is why when we do a traditional Lomi session for healing, we use our breath over the body to do away with the old and purify the memory of the muscle to become clear. The "Ha" breath would be beneficial for anybody to learn.

The Kupuna always knew the benefit of true healing from the heart. Their ancient knowledge has been carried into today for all to know and learn whenever anyone is ready. Fortunately, my expansion of knowledge was just about to take another leap when Papa K introduced me to Pele, the fire Goddess of Hawaii.

~ Beautiful Pele ~

If you ever have heard of the Goddess Pele, the legend is tremendous. She is known as the Kilauea Volcano in Hilo, on the Big Island of Hawaii. Thousands of people flock to the island to see her luscious lava pour into the ocean as well as to enjoy the beauty and peace in a land of enchantment. It is said that if you take a lava rock from her without asking, your life will have many significant reactions that are not positive experiences! This is true.

When I was studying with my Kupuna, he used to tell me that Pele's love was like a precious grandmother (which is where she developed the name "Tutu Pele"). I saw that he had a great affiliation to her personality, and this fascinated me. There is a center at the Volcano National Park where people return stones because their lives had gone awry. This just made me more excited about meeting Pele. The Kupuna had mentioned that when you come home to Hawaii, Pele gets very happy to have her grandchild back. It does not matter if it's this life or one where she knew you before. The feeling I had when I first laid eyes on her was unlike any feeling I had ever experienced.

One day, the Kupuna was having trouble physically. I knew I could work with him to do a great healing. However, he was plagued with diabetes and had a recent operation in which he lost his leg. So I went to the Volcano National Park and spoke to Pele. Much to my surprise, she and I developed an instant love for each other, and she began to blow wind my way. It got undeniably strong. My inner voice was calm and I began to listen. I started hearing words in the wind. (SO THIS is what the Native Americans mean when we "listen to the wind!") She told me to go back and tell the Kupuna that he must act within the laws of Aloha. "True to Self" is the term we use, called "Pono." She told me a few things I didn't even read as an energy runner. I was surprised yet also relieved that I could go back and tell him. He heard it.

Well, this became rather addicting to know that I could tune in and hear her when she wanted to talk to me. When Pele is listening to your request and accepts your gifts of flowers or fruit, she will show as a white bird going solo in the crater. She flies so magnificently that you cannot help but know the grace of her beauty.

So I went back once a week for one year, expressing my love through chanting, singing (mele), and listening to her marvelous wisdom. I left to come back to the mainland after my training was complete on October 14, 2006. On the morning before I went to say goodbye, the fumes of the vog (volcano fog) were beginning to get strong. On October 13th, early in the morning, I looked out over the crater and realized something was not right. The bird did not show.

I waited about 15 minutes and told Pele that I refused to leave until I saw the bird and knew she was alright. Two minutes passed, and the bird flew sideways in the crater. She had shown herself, but then something strange happened! The bird disappeared right before my eyes. It was there, and then it was gone. I waited a few minutes, and she reappeared, again doing the same. I realized I was stubborn, but this was Pele's way of telling me it was time to go. I had to make sure she was all right. Yet because Pele is all about respect, I listened and walked away with a sad heart.

It was the hardest thing I had ever done, but I knew I would be back when it was time. Pele would call me in my heart. I knew that I would feel it. Midnight came, and I was on a plane back to the West Coast. I was traveling with a dear friend. Before we entered the plane, I looked at her and said, "If 9/11 had happened here, would you still call this Paradise??" We boarded right after that.

I arrived to my destination six hours later to hear the televisions in the airport blurting out loud that there was a 6.6 earthquake on the Big Island of Hawaii at 7 a.m. on October 14th.

The time came when I returned to see Pele on October 14, 2009, not realizing that it had been three years to the day since that last visit. I went back because a client gave me a 10-day stay to write this book on Maui. Yet I knew I was being "called" to go alone. I made it my retreat and spent the last four days in Hilo and Kona. I finally got to see Pele the last day I was on the Island. I knew something was up because the call was strong.

When I arrived at the Volcano National Park, I was right. Holding the orchids I had to give Pele, I got out of the car in the parking lot and fell straight down to my knees with the hardest grief I had ever experienced! I cried so spontaneously, it was like projectile vomiting. When I picked myself up and walked over to the crater, I noticed my heart pouring love (ALOHA) and felt as though I had never left her.

My heart was saddened, however, because the grief I was feeling clearly was not mine but hers. I sat next to the crater and told Pele I was there to help in any way I could. She then showed me the beautiful white bird! The shine radiating from the wings was enough to soften that sad feeling. This was a reunion.

Then the wind blew. I consider this the "Ha" breath, so I blew back to her. She had me listen to the message that she needed (and wanted) me to share. This message abides today, and so I share it with you. She asked me to put her in the book.

Here is her message:

"Seven hundred and fifty thousand people have come to see me since you left me three years ago today. In that 750,000, not one has seen me. Their fear is great. They are afraid that the vog is hurting them. They are afraid of the volcano blowing up and then killing them. They look the other way when a lesson comes up for them to learn.

I pour myself into that Ocean for the people so they can create this new land with the Aloha Spirit originally intended and bring back a land that is fresh, new, and expansive. If the people knew that this is why the lava flows now, maybe they would add their true hearts of simplicity, gratitude, and love. But they are too busy speaking of Atlantis and Lemuria. Those places became corrupt. Why do you think I buried them?"

Fear of making changes and fear of losing a life seem to be the highlight here. Our conversations were "in the flow" of hearing each other when at that time, this connection of dialogue was crucial. It wasn't an eruption of lava from her that was the issue. It was the eruption of fear in the people that was necessary for me. It was the understanding I was to comprehend as a conduit with and FOR her.

This important message I just shared with you was overwhelming for me at that moment. So that explained why I was called to listen and cry with her at that time! Now if we can hear that message today and humble to the knowledge that fear was based in ego…not Spirit…then we can start to live differently within our hearts with less fear all together.

Permission and respect are of utmost importance in Hawaii and everywhere else on Earth. When taking a lava rock, as long as you ask permission, and you do it with love, then it becomes a gift of the land to you. The honored respect in which giving and receiving occur is the balance of the land and the people being one. Pele pours graciousness and peace in her lava flow. We need to pay attention. With fear, not only do we find ourselves blocking deeper connections but also we resist the highest form of love one could possibly have.

~ The Connection ~

The quantum aspect of healing is allowing a change in our belief systems with respect to knowledge that we haven't learned yet. Knowing that there is always more makes us feel as though we are like new babies with potentials and dynamic abilities we haven't even touched. How exciting to realize that one shifted perception can change the world. I know this is a lot to comprehend. However, if you consider that quantum thought has no time, then that leaves the door wide open for possibilities.

This, then, is how we continue to move forward in a world by contributing to it, not being run by it. As Jesus so eloquently phrased it, "I am in the world, not of it." Being in higher frequencies, we can now say we are almost ready as a collective unit in this school of humanity to be in it *and* of it as our consciousness rises as a whole. Whether we understand it or not, we are becoming a collective in the realm of quantum thought and instant manifestation. I feel so inspired when I remember the stories of Christ. I do feel that this is what Jesus's purpose was from the beginning. Who knows? Maybe this IS the second coming, the Christ Consciousness in action!

My recently deceased business partner, John Jay Harper, loved going on the radio to share his insights into the future, and people loved his sweet voice of wisdom. He wrote the following paragraph for a new book he had been writing:

> "When we look through the lens of microscopes and telescopes, we see there are no boundaries to creation. We are a soup. Thus, in the final analysis, we are not and cannot be separate from each other, nature, or God. There is only one source of intelligence underlying reality that we call the vacuum of space, or the zero-point field. The implication is that we are immortal beings of light that come and go, lifetime after lifetime, through a membrane made of consciousness itself."

As 2012 continues to unfold, we are being given a gift. This is the time of change, of fortune, of unraveling the past. We are seeing our issues brought up in order to release them.

On a personal note, I feel this is the best year ever. It is the true beginning of our future of interpersonal relationships with like-minded people to create a unity of conscious teamwork. Even better, we are creating a community of people who are mastering their love for each other by living directly from their hearts.

The heart of the matter is truly the matter of the heart.

This is the wave of the future by terms of the Indigenous and by terms of Science. With organizations such as HeartMath, Director Howard Martin teaches us the direct magnification of our human heart and the connection to the Earth, the Solar Flares, and each other. We have no reason to discount this epic opportunity to unite.

What is the difference, then, in Indigenous concepts and understandings vs. scientific facts and comprehension? They are one and the same. There is no difference. However, the energy force that drives a Shaman to that knowledge is gratitude and recognition of conscious oneness. That leads to wisdom and gracious humility. That then will lead to happiness so our cells know that through our shifting, we are one with all things. Energy runs our world. We can transmute anything and everything.

According to some Native American traditions, this is known as "snake medicine." We are learning that we are shedding our old skin (patterns, thoughts, limited belief systems, etc.) on a personal and global level. Now if we can combine that knowledge with the knowing of *where two or more are gathered*, we will then see that the energy of one is one, two is two hundred, three is three thousand, and so on.

Truthfully, this is how we can change the world together and recreate the bountiful and once luscious planet, Heaven on Earth.

In the eyes of a Shaman, we feel *connected* to all things. We respect the land, our tribe and mostly, our Selves. Without that we might as well not be Shamans. When we speak of raising Consciousness we are really saying that our internal world must be whole and complete, as we know we cannot sufficiently live without nature. You might say we become a Universe within ourselves and create a harmonic frequency when we do this together. This alone initializes peace and oneness, and that brings about more peace and oneness.

Quantum facts are not judgments. They are precisely correct and can change any amount of energy in seconds. Energy healing can be better understood from this way of viewing. This is why it is so important to understand that our perceptions are mutable and can change an entire planet from being in chaos and separation to being all related and united.

8.

THE GALACTIC HUMAN

"We are literally thought forms co-existing within the mind of God. If we apply this eternal Truth to our lives, we can peacefully co-exist with all life forms. This eternal Truth stands here and hereafter..." - John Jay Harper

We are at a time of dramatic change, not only in ourselves, but in the world and even in the Universe. Most of us have already discovered that these changes are affecting the ways we live, think, and make decisions, which formerly were based on concepts we figured had been working for us. With major economic changes alone, we are questioning what's next for the Global Community as well as for our own families. The "Clarion Call" for awakening to awareness in 2012 is advancing at an unprecedented rate. Yet the feeling of change is light, and the drifting away of our old ways of living and thinking is allowing us to be free of our past, both individually and through our behaviors globally. We are doing this in the form of *Consciousness*.

In the book, *The Gaia Project*, written by Hwee-Yong Jang and translated by Mira Tyson, it states that "Consciousness can be defined as a faculty of a being who perceives the world and creates something out of that perception. From this viewpoint, the nature of being, including that of the human beings, can be described as consciousness."

I love that definition of Consciousness, mainly because it indicates that perception is the guiding force of where we lead ourselves and gives new meaning to the phrase "*As within, so without.*" The conscious brain sits in our prefrontal cortex. It is responsible for our creativity and has no perception of time. It doesn't hang onto our personal identity and is capable of shifting reality into non-reality. Actually, it is what really gives us empowerment...or not.

The vast intelligence of the Universe lives inside of each and every one of us. It awaits that recognition once again so we may be transformed by it. We simply could not have this in us if we didn't already understand it on some level. Science has proven over and over again that the cells have more space than they do matter. Therefore, enlarging our knowledge and ability to become more than we *think* we are will expand and do away with our limited concepts. By opening our minds and allowing these new downloaded insights to take effect, it is like "Sa-hae-lu" in the movie Avatar. The connection to our cosmic self begins to take hold inside of our very cells. We are waking up in awareness, self confidence, and many more wonderful adventures of manifestation. The beauty of living on this planet requires a oneness of these attributes.

The encouragements of these new acknowledgments are taking place within us through simple experiences now, such as: Wiggling your toes in the sand. Going barefoot and feeling the cool grass engaging your feet in its pleasure to laugh along with you. Being silent and sitting in the stillness of a forest. Hearing the sounds of a loud gushing waterfall piercing your senses to be recognized, making its presence known.

This doesn't need a lot of explanation, just the simple awareness that these beautiful gifts of nature are here to be included always. Simplicity is the way of the Shaman. It is always about the connection. Therefore, when we hear the sayings, "We are all one" or "We are all family", it's that connection to truth that sets us into a freedom of the moment.

Soon we will be encountering more of what our planets are helping our brains to wake up to and comprehend. No longer will it be that our beliefs run our lives. We may find that we have no beliefs whatsoever. Pure consciousness IS about living in the moment. Beliefs can stifle that moment, consciously or subconsciously, until we are awakened by an experience that blows all of the old expectations out the window. In our times today in 2012, life is about to give us back our Selves, without any pretense.

The subconscious mind is in the rest of the brain and lives in the present moment. It doesn't understand creation the way the conscious mind does because it identifies itself as the big picture. We minimize this and turn it into *creation* through the conscious mind. That is what makes us co-creators in the vastness of life itself. It is what gives us our personal choices in order to live in a way we can understand. The subconscious doesn't see the same way the conscious does, so this is where we can become more aware of our personal contribution to life.

~ John Jay Harper's
Last Message for the World ~

My business partner in 2010, John Jay Harper, was an Author, a Scientist, and a Visionary. On December 11, 2010, he was asked to be a guest on a radio program from Australia. In this part of the chapter, I am including his wisdom from that show that he so intended to share more of. John left this world on the 15th of December, only four days after the interview was broadcast to the world.

John was one of the most passionate men I have ever met, a true genius when it came to understanding Life, Love, God, the Polar Shift, and the Human Race. He was author of *Transformers: Shamans of the 21st Century*. I wasn't aware of his book at all when I met him. Actually, I had no idea he was an author at all. When we met, not only did I find out that he was an author of this marvelous book, but I also found out that he had been on the internet on several blog talk radio shows as well as Coast to Coast.

We met one day (quite spontaneously) on Facebook. He sought help for a condition in his neck that he thought was from a car accident forty years prior. His ears rang relentlessly, and the pain in his neck was indescribable. He had tried all of the alternative methods for help and had resorted to medical drug therapy, which didn't work, either. Nothing he had found was able to relieve the ringing or the pain.

He invited me to his home in Spokane, Washington, where I met his wife, daughter, and grandchildren. The day I met John at the airport, we felt as though we had always known each other. Therefore, I enjoyed my three-day stays in July and again in August of 2010. I had explained my work to John before I met him. I told him I could energetically read him, his past, and even his thoughts. Over the phone, he saw that this was true. This was why I originally went to his home.

Our hearts became very connected as close friends and (agreed upon) business partners. Our very connection alone was magnificent. As energy proves not to know distance, we had a shared death experience. Author Raymond Moody explains in his book, *Life after Life*, "A shared death experience is stronger than a near death experience for the one left behind." I can certainly attest to that! Spiritual experiences are happening more and more as time gets stronger in the new paradigm of living.

John wasn't afraid of passing at all. His fascination with NDE's (near-death experiences) continued to expand as he himself was getting ready for the next adventure.

His writings on the topic of health were fresh, clear, and insightful. They included quotes from many authors, including Joseph Campbell, author of *The Power of Myth* and *An Open Life*. He enjoyed quoting the Bible and also musical artists. He quoted Huey Lewis and the News singing, "We need a new drug, one that won't make us sick." He and I spoke of Humanity needing to wake up to what real health was all about. It was something we were both willing to share together in the world.

We were the Scientist and the Shaman coming together to teach how to upgrade our DNA software file codes and brain hardware circuits for life in the 21st Century. Now that John is gone, I am moved to abide by his request and write the book that has been inside me throughout my entire life. We both made an agreement that everything we did together would be 50/50. This partnership ranged from talks, books, and CD's to radio programs, which we planned to begin in February, 2011. Now I include his awesome information in this book to keep my end of the bargain.

Many people on Facebook and friends and family were looking forward to our work. Yes, I must say, we had a knack for sharing insights.

After John had passed, his wife Connie generously asked me to go through John's information and take what I felt pertinent to share with the world. I collaborated with what his best writings and teachings entailed and put together what he would have wanted all of us to know from his scientific and visionary understandings for 2012 and beyond.

Some of what I am about to share is also about the Earth and the lead-in to the current Polar Shift we are now experiencing. Keep in mind that John wasn't here on this planet in 2011. I will point out that he wanted everyone to understand the importance of living at heart center. We both taught this, similar to what we hear now with HeartMath, Gregg Braden, and many other wonderful teachers in our world. Our future existence is and will be more based directly from our hearts. We will think from our heart center as we feel answers merge with the thoughts as an after-effect. The mind makes a terrible employer but does very well as an employee of the heart.

~ A Holographic Projection ~

Because John was a scientist in all of his great understandings of facts and knowledge, I loved asking him questions. One sunny afternoon on his deck, we were enjoying a conversation about holograms. I asked him if his idea of a hologram was different from the dictionary's, mainly because the dictionary was brief. (I chuckle here because John was anything but brief!) He said that the word *"hologram"* meant, *whole message*. The whole is in the part, and the part is in the whole. So when it came to discussing Universal facts, he said the Universe is actually a holographic projection.

From a personal standpoint, the hologram is the way we see through our mind's eye (the 3rd eye). Holography, then, is the way the brain processes electromagnetic information through the nervous system, which creates images in the brain. We convert a signal of information into an image, and this is how we perceive life.

We live in a multi-dimensional reality. Everything that can exist does exist. We seem to be tuned to a **human** perception of reality. This can make things seem strange if we don't understand, for example, why we have dreams that don't make sense. It's what is called the *bleed through* of other dimensions seeping into our personal consciousness. From other realities, we are able to tap into dreamtime.

The Shaman knows that dreamtime is sacred and respected as a way of communication from Spirit for our highest good. We wouldn't be tapping into something so magnificent and vast unless we had the capacity to expand, and on some level, to understand this in our own consciousness. Therefore, our dreams are real. We know this from waking up with a sense of realism from another world. So, as John described, in order to make something real, either consciously or subconsciously, we would have to mentally allow willpower to play a part in this. (Now here's where it gets a little scientific, but I'll explain it in layman's terms in the best way to understand what is happening today.)

This introduces the concept and reality of *magnetics*. We're talking about ley lines and song lines, grid lines in the earth which are similar to meridians of the physical body. Magnetics draw out to what is like it and can vibrate at the same capacity. Now that we are kicking up more vibrations of the electromagnetic field, our minds are expanding. We are going into the zero-point fields. This simply put means that we are about to start a new cycle of time and have a choice on how that will be done. We will begin to tap into these multi-dimensional realms much more as time continues.

Even now we are talking about seeing angels, aliens, loved ones who have crossed, all in our scope of vision. As time continues, the realms will also include more lucid dreaming. We actually may feel drawn to a place when we wake back into *this* world, and this world will seem like the one that is *not* real. I hear people talking a lot about this today. So it seems that this is true in the times we are living.

Since we are tuning into too many frequencies at once, this may not feel *normal* to us anymore. The typical human being isn't used to all of this energy elevation. If we tune into this *bleed through*, we are going to create a perception of reality that is not going to match our neighbor, family members, et al. This would be considered *abnormal* by today's standards. It's time that we begin to practice "abnormal physics and paranormal psychology!"

~ Who Are We? ~

"Our pineal gland is becoming activated. We need to unload our minds, realizing we are becoming impeccably aware that we are all leaders, teachers, and students." - John Jay Harper

First of all, when we realize how much alike we are yet so individually unique, we have to see that life is actually comical in its simplicity. Now we can find ourselves giggling at the idea of judgment because we are feeling that there is no need for this type of primitive thinking, either within ourselves or in the world. Unfortunately, even though we see it continuing to occur around different parts of the world, our knowledge of this type of thinking supports the fact that judgment is losing its false power. Therefore, we will not pay heed to such a low vibration.

We are rising above the mundane as time continues to help us acknowledge the truth of our oneness. On one of John's last radio interviews, he was asked the question, "Who are we?" His eloquent style and passion proved to be profound once again when his answer stated:

"We are a species now that is developing
into a multi- dimensional consciousness. We are
an experiment in consciousness, if you will, and
are going into a field of cosmic consciousness.
This means that we are going into our hearts.
What the human being is doing now is waking
up. We are holding hands together as we walk
into this new level of reality.

We are transducers, transmitters and
receivers of consciousness that is generated
by the Earth, by our Solar System, and by
the center of the Galaxy. We are really in a
window of opportunity for the human being
to tune into this Galactic Center.

This sense of unity, or *at-one-ment*, with the cosmos shows us that time seems to be speeding up. For some, it is slowing down. For others, it has stopped, and we are coming into the moment of the eternal NOW that the mystics have taught us for centuries. As we become increasingly activated in this process, we will increase our awareness. We now are beginning to feel more as we *feel* our way into the future individually and collectively."

He continued to discuss eco-location, the way that dolphins process information in their environment in the ocean: "They send a signal, as we know, and they take that information as it comes off an object and is returned to their consciousness. They create an image of that. It becomes holographic in their communication."

As John continued to impress the radio host, he added many other wonderful insights as to where we are going in this newfound state of aligned consciousness with and of the Universe. He talked about the idea of telepathy that was initially a sense of mind-to-mind communication. With that said, intuition will then become a visual image. We are feeling our way into the future because the signal now is low, but as we link up with this in our minds (our mind's eye, the third eye) through the pineal gland, this image will become stronger and stronger. It will be a sense of actually turning ourselves inside out. The outside and the inside will become one side. We will see new skills coming our way.

~ Awakening the Planetary Mind ~

Now that we are recognizing the changes on the planet and within ourselves, many of us are feeling a strange sense of emptiness or a sense of *disconnect* to who we used to be. As scary as this feels, it is right in line with the waking up process. In other words, as we let go of the old ideas of our identity, we are feeling our way in through a new awareness.

Recently many people have been afraid that they are going crazy. Our thinking is being challenged because a strong sense of our future will not be led by *thinking* as we've known it. The thinking process will align with heart-centered living, and as we become more active in this state, we will begin to realize that our thoughts are like monkey chatter. Therefore, we will be able consciously to quiet our minds much better and to move forward without associated fears getting in the way.

One way to see these fears is to realize that certain conditions of the physical body are taking effect faster and faster as manifestation occurs at a quicker rate. Some people are being diagnosed with bipolar disorder. Several types of personality disorders are also being diagnosed. Our stress levels are becoming higher the more we try to live the way we always have thought we needed to in order to survive in this world.

It can take us out of our comfort zones as we live in the challenge of change. As negative as it may seem, it isn't at all. It is the perception that unfamiliarity creates emptiness and a fear. Some people then react to this fear by negative behavior, guilt, shame, anger, and blame. If you have noticed these within you, just know that all of the behavior patterns within us that have not been dealt with are being amplified.

NOW is the time to recognize that we can choose to change. Old primitive concepts are definitely a thing of the past as we launch into new awareness. This brings with it opportunity beyond our conscious understanding and what some would term as "magic" that is basically a form of alignment to the new creation we are becoming, individually and collectively.

Many people are talking about a Polar Shift happening today and for the next few years. If we read Gregg Braden's book *Deep Truth*, we will see that he has depicted cycles that have been occurring on our planet and in the Solar System for thousands of years. He states, "We appeared on Earth, looking as we do today, 200,000 years, ---30 world-age cycles and two ice ages ago." He tells us that our bodies bear the unmistakable signs of an intelligent design. This we know from eons of time being here on Earth, so now we need to awaken the process more into this intelligence through the understanding of our real, true power.

Planets, just like us, have recurring patterns as they rotate and offer another go around. However, we are now in a conscious position of being able to align with this particular timing and change. Our loving Universe gives us the encouragement with the momentum of *full speed ahead*. Instead of resisting our Divine Intelligence, maybe this time we can understand. Oneness occurring in this cycle can change our present 3rd dimensional living into a 5th dimensional awareness of Divine interaction into freedom.

Consciousness or Spirit is a magnetic phenomenon. Living in the physical body alone doesn't make sense when we know now that we are the driver of our body through our thoughts, mental creativity, and perceptions of our own realities. This is why so many authors of NDE's (near-death experiences) are enjoying teaching us and describing the death process as a phenomenon of feeling, such as being pulled out of the body like a magnetic iron filing.

Even the Law of Attraction is a magnetic phenomenon. Likes attract; opposites repel. So where we are now, and where we are continuing to go, is magnetic in itself. When electricity and magnetics unite, we have an electromagnetic occurrence. Our Solar flares today are enhancing this effect within us, individually and collectively, and helping the old to become new. Therefore, knowing that a Pole Shift is occurring helps us to realize that it is an electromagnetic shift that is bringing back the electrical and magnetic components of the Earth, which is opening the floodgates of consciousness.

It is crucial for unity, for Oneness, to be understood and lived. We are a human race given all potential to be one unit, to work as one unit, to achieve splendor in our hearts and souls. It is imperative now to accept this ultimate blessing and to change the world. Now is our time to shine like never before and utilize the astrological abundance being offered.

Humanity is becoming shamanized.

In John Jay Harper's words, "We are becoming conscious now of being co-creators of a new heaven and a new earth. Whatever we can create, we can manifest.

Whatever we can create, we *will* manifest!"

~ My Conclusion ~

There are seven billion people on this Earth today. All of us are here for a reason. Does that mean we have to get hung up on a purpose? Author and lecturer, Joseph Campbell, was asked several years ago about the word "purpose" in the interview with Bill Moyer. His answer was this: "We ask ourselves if we have a purpose in this world. My suggestion is to do away with that word because it continues to demean why we are here to begin with."

If we realize that being here on the planet is fulfilling a purpose in itself, maybe we won't think we are wasting our time here or wonder if we should even be here. If you converse with someone, show a smile, laugh, or even enjoy your God-given life, you can rest assured that you have done something to change the way things are today.

What is important is not just feeling purpose but actually having a willingness to keep your heart open. The heart is the magnet and the reflector. My desire is to help enlighten people to their health, which is the natural state of the human body. No matter where we are, energy is the ticket to anything we want to see different. Even if we are on another planet, the key is still energy.

I personally ask you to give this information I have shared with you a chance. Own it, breathe it, live it even in the midst of a challenging shift. In doing so, you will change your old patterns through this acceptance. As you begin to feel that everything has a purpose and a reason, you will help change our world.

When our hearts speak, the whole world hears it.

I love you dearly, each and every one of you. Thank you for being here, and thank you for reading this book for your continued journey into your newfound joy.

Notes:

CPSIA information can be obtained at www.ICGtesting.com
Printed in the USA
LVOW05s1458160214

373892LV00023B/1201/P